Clinicians' Guide to *Helicobacter pylori*

Clinicians' Guide to
Helicobacter pylori

John Calam MD FRCP

Reader in Gastroenterology
Hammersmith Hospital
London

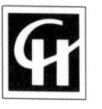
CHAPMAN & HALL MEDICAL
London · Weinheim · New York · Tokyo · Melbourne · Madras

Published by Chapman & Hall, 2-6 Boundary Row, London SE1 8HN, UK

Chapman & Hall, 2-6 Boundary Row, London SE1 8HN, UK

Chapman & Hall GmbH, Pappelallee 3, 69469 Weinheim, Germany

Chapman & Hall USA, 115 Fifth Avenue, New York, NY 10003, USA

Chapman & Hall Japan, ITP-Japan, Kyowa Building, 3F, 2–2–1 Hirakawacho, Chiyoda-ku, Tokyo 102, Japan

Chapman & Hall Australia, 102 Dodds Street, South Melbourne, Victoria 3205, Australia

Chapman & Hall India, R. Seshadri, 32 Second Main Road, CIT East, Madras 600 035, India

First edition 1996
Reprinted 1996

© 1996 John Calam

Typeset in 11/12½ pt Palatino by WestKey Ltd, Falmouth, Cornwall
Printed in Great Britain at the University Press, Cambridge
ISBN 0 412 74000 1

A catalogue record for this book is available from the British Library

Library of Congress Catalog Card Number: 95-79871

∞ Printed on permanent acid-free text paper, manufactured in accordance with ANSI/NISO Z39.48-1992 and ANSI/NISO Z39.48-1984 (Permanence of Paper).

Contents

Preface

It has been exciting to witness the discovery that most peptic ulcers are caused by a bacterium that is relatively easy to eradicate. Most doctors now aim to give their patients the benefits of this unexpected breakthrough, but the new knowledge raises many questions. One is precisely which groups of patients to treat. We should restrict ourselves to the infected, but which of the many tests should we use to identify them? Having decided to treat, which of the plethora of regimens should we use? These questions have been particularly difficult to address at a time when knowledge and clinical techniques are still developing rapidly.

This book aims to present the current scene in an objective and digestible form, so that clinicians can choose strategies which suit their local needs. The relative merits of the various clinical approaches are discussed, together with some scientific background to prepare the reader for future developments. The book is primarily aimed at practising clinicians but should be equally useful for students preparing for examinations. It will also provide a source of reference to workers in the pharmaceutical industry, journalism or marketing who need to get 'up-to-speed' in this area.

One key question is why *H. pylori* causes different diseases in different people. The answer will hopefully indicate who to treat first! Therefore, discussion of bacteriology includes an outline of the toxic bacterial products, and the important finding that some strains are more pathogenic than others. Spread of *H. pylori* seems to be mainly faecal–oral and the diseases that it causes become less prevalent when hygiene improves. The chapter on disease associations also addresses pathogenic mechanisms, and includes conditions, such as non-ulcer dyspepsia, whose relationship with *H. pylori* remains unclear. Diagnostic methods are described in some detail to assist the choice of test, which includes low-cost 'in-house' methods.

The accuracy of the tests varies and some require local validation. Discussion of eradication regimens highlights the best available but also indicates why previous recipes were rejected. The discovery of *H. pylori* has led to a complete rethink of clinical strategies. Flow charts are included but clinical assessment remains vital. The final chapter looks into the future, in the expectation that developments will lead to further improvements in clinical management.

I gratefully acknowledge the help and advice given by my many expert colleagues. These include Professor Adrian Lee, Professor Robert Feldman, Dr Michael Dixon, Dr Peter Sullivan, Dr Erik Rauws, Professor Gabiele Bianchi Porro, Professor Francis Megraud, Professor David Forman, Dr Adam Harris and Dr George Misiewicz, whose excellent reviews are cited in the relevant chapters. I also thank colleagues who have advised on the diagnostic techniques that they have developed, as well as Dr Ashley Price and others who have provided illustrations. We all admire the pioneering work of Robin Warren and Barry Marshall, whose efforts have enriched our medical and scientific activities and helped our patients. On a personal note, I thank my wife Joyce for her patience and support while I was writing this book.

John Calam, London

1

Discovery and bacteriology

INTRODUCTION

It has been quite a shock to the system to discover that several of the gastroduodenal diseases that we thought we understood fairly well are actually caused by a bacterium; *Helicobacter pylori*. This book aims to explore the clinical implications of this remarkable discovery. But before we do – why didn't someone discover this earlier? The question is worth asking because the answer might indicate how modern science can still discover the unexpected. Clearly we were looking in the wrong direction. Most of our minds were fixed on two simple concepts:

- The stomach secretes acid to keep it sterile.
- Too much acid causes ulcers.

Major laboratories, by their nature, pursue conventional ideas in great detail. Pharmaceutical companies and peer-reviewed grant-awarding bodies prefer to support elegant studies of more-or-less conventional ideas. In this case the companies did so brilliantly: histamine H_2-antagonists were developed by Black and his colleagues at Smith Kline and French in 1972 [1]. The H^+/K^+ ATPase inhibitor omeprazole was first synthesized by the team at Astra Sweden in 1979. The first report of its effect in humans appeared in *Gut* in 1981 [2]. In the next year *H. pylori* was first cultured by a research registrar, Marshall, encouraged by a histopathologist, Warren, in Perth, Australia. The message is clear: we do need medical academics, and part of their role is to play the 'mad scientist' and explore the unconventional ideas that larger scientific organizations shun.

EARLY SIGHTINGS

Bottcher reported the presence of spiral organisms in the stomachs of mammals over 120 years ago in 1874 [3]. By 1900 this had been confirmed by others, and Salomon had shown that the spiral bacterium which infects dogs and cats can be transmitted to mice [4]. This phenomenon is currently used in the development of immunization against helicobacters. Spiral bacteria were first seen in the human stomach by Kreinitz in 1906 [5] and two further reports had appeared by the end of 1940. These reports showed, remarkably, that about 40% of human stomachs contained the spirochaetes. So far, all of this work had taken place in Europe. Unfortunately the first study in America poured cold water on the whole idea. Palmer reported in *Gastroenterology* in 1954 that he was unable to find the bacteria in suction biopsies from 1180 human stomachs [6]!

Another line of evidence emerged in 1924 when Luck and Seth reported that the human stomach contains abundant urease activity [7]. It was shown in 1959 that this activity disappeared during administration of antibiotics, indicating that the enzyme is of bacterial origin. However the connection between gastric urease and gastric spiral bacteria was not made until 1984 [8].

At this stage progress was blocked by general disbelief and also by an inability to culture the bacteria. In 1975 Steer reported spiral bacteria closely applied to gastric-mucus-secreting cells in the human stomach, but culture only yielded *Pseudomonas aeruginosa* [9].

THE FIRST CULTURE

H. pylori was first cultured in Perth, Western Australia. Early reports from that centre were not encouraging. Fung observed by light and electron microscopy that the bacteria did not invade epithelial cells, and concluded that they were not pathogenic [10]. Despite this, Warren maintained his interest in the bacteria and made the important observation that most patients with gastritis or ulcers were infected with curved or *Campylobacter*-like organisms [11]. Therefore he encouraged Marshall to try to culture the bacteria from endoscopic biopsies, using methods for the culture of campylobacters which had become available by that time. Culture for the usual period of 48 hours produced no growth. The first successful culture occurred by serendipity when the 35th biopsy was left in the incubator for 5 days over the Easter holidays in April 1982! Marshall accepted and developed Warren's idea that the infection was associated with gastritis, and with duodenal and gastric ulcers [12]. In 1984 Rollason, Stone and Rhodes [13] in Selly Oak Hospital, Birmingham, and Steer [14] in Southampton General Hospital also reported that patients with gastritis or ulcers were infected with the spiral bacteria more often than healthy controls. Thus three groups had independently reported the main disease associations of *H. pylori*. Marshall thought that the new bacteria was a *Campylobacter* found in the pyloric region of the stomach and therefore called it *Campylobacter pyloridis*. *Pyloridis* became *pylori* when linguists pointed out that the former was grammatically incorrect. *Campylobacter* became *Helicobacter* when it was discovered that its 16S ribosomal RNA did not have the characteristic sequences found in campylobacters [15]. A new genus had been discovered!

BACTERIOLOGICAL FEATURES

H. pylori is a spiral or curved microaerophilic Gram-negative rod, equipped with 4–6 flagellae at one end [15] (Figures 1.1 and 1.2). Bacterial products which are believed to contribute to disease processes are described in this chapter, and also in Chapter 3. However, the bacterium's unique feature is its ability to colonize the stomach. To do so *H. pylori* has to cope with gastric acid, as well as the gastric immune response.

Adaptation to the acid milieu

Gastric acid kills most bacteria but gastric helicobacters have evolved some special features which allow them to live in this acidic niche.

Induction of a lack of acid during first attack
When *H. pylori* first infects the stomach it induces a profound lack of acid secretion which lasts for several months after first infection [16]. Researchers who used the same tube to measure acid secretion in different people found that some subjects developed vague upper gastrointestinal symptoms and ceased to secrete acid. Retrospective analysis of sera from these individuals showed that this 'epidemic achlorhydria' was actually due to first infections with *H. pylori*. The infection was presumably transmitted between the subjects by the gastric tube, which was not disinfected because the stomach was thought to be sterile! Two mechanisms have been

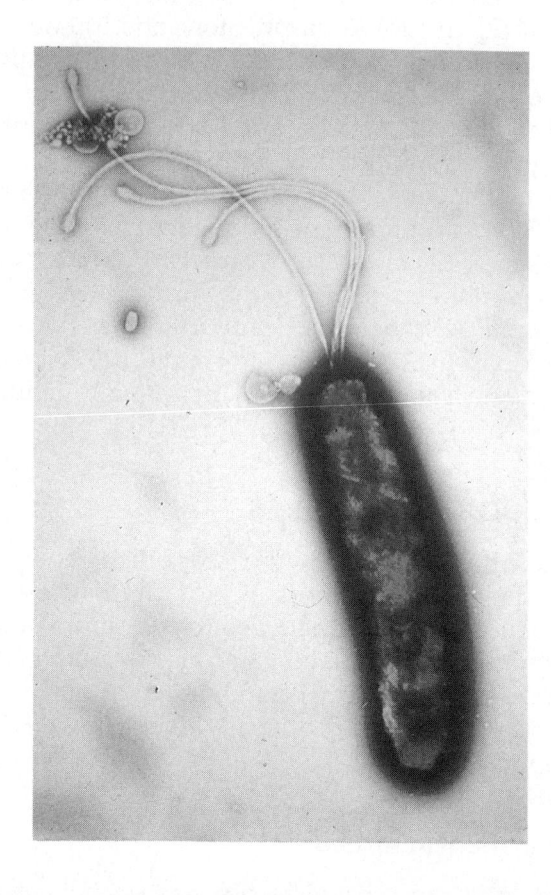

Figure 1.1 Electron micrograph (EM) of *Helicobacter pylori* showing its curved shape and flagellae. Photo: Heather Davies/Chapman & Hall/SPL

proposed for the loss of acid secretion. Firstly *H. pylori* releases at least one product which stops parietal cells from producing acid [17]. Secondly interleukin-1, which is released by leucocytes in *H. pylori* gastritis, inhibits acid secretion when injected into rats [18]. In this context it is interesting that histamine-fast achlorhydria also occurs during other infections such as typhoid, paratyphoid, pulmonary tuberculosis, bronchopneumonia and lung abscess. This was reported from a region of China which has a low natural incidence of achlorhydria [19]. Whatever the mechanism, the lack of acid secretion may help *H. pylori* to become established in the stomach.

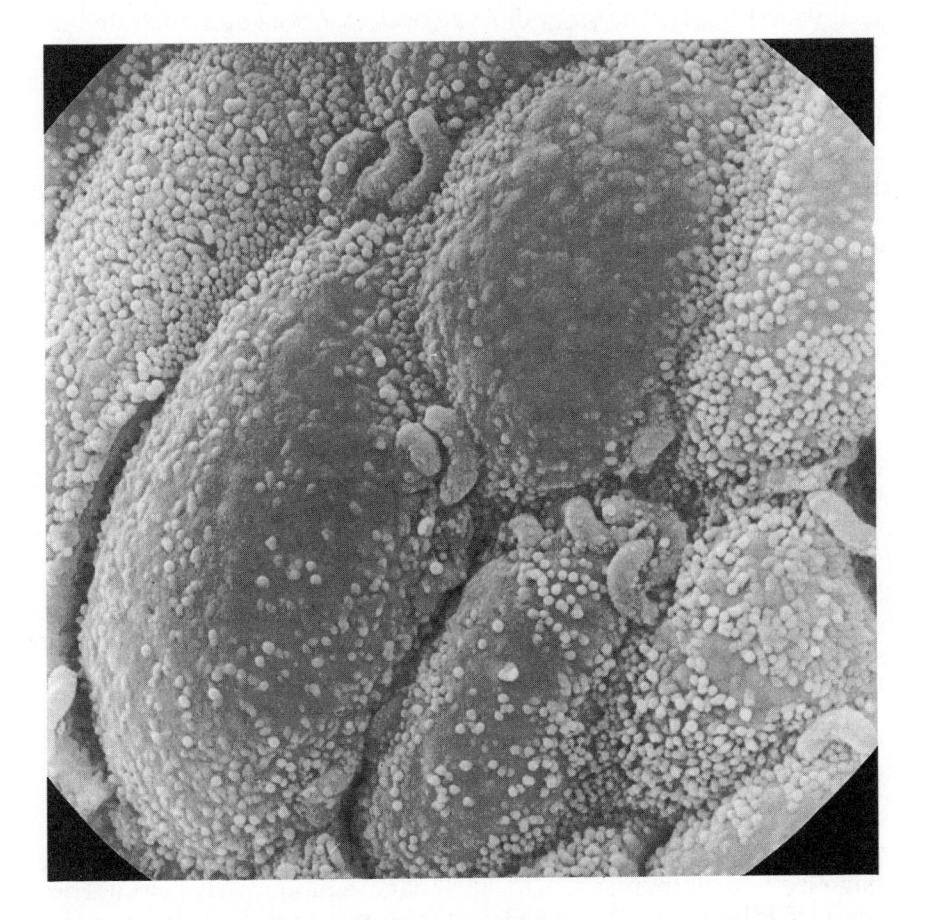

Figure 1.2 Scanning electron micrograph showing *Helicobacter pylori* bacteria on the surface of the gastric epithelium. Courtesy of Dr M. Walker.

Urease
Urea diffuses freely from plasma into gastric juice. *H. pylori* produces large amounts of the nickel-containing enzyme [20] urease, which digests urea to produce one carbon dioxide and two ammonia molecules, leading to net production of alkali.

$$NH_2–CO–NH_2 + H_2O \rightarrow CO_2 + 2NH_3$$

Then spontaneously at neutral pH:

$$NH_3 + H_2O \rightarrow NH_4OH \rightarrow NH_4^+ + OH^-.$$

Without urea *H. pylori* are intolerant of acid, but in its presence the bacterium prefers mildly acidic conditions and can withstand a pH as low as 1.5 [21]. The essential role of urease was demonstrated in gnotobiotic piglets (i.e. piglets with a defined bacterial flora). Wild-type *H. pylori* colonized these animals but a strain that lacked urease did not [22]. Gastric juice from patients with *H. pylori* infection contains less urea and more ammonium ions than normal. Indeed the infection could be diagnosed by measuring urea and ammonium ions in the patient's gastric juice [23], if there were no better methods. From the clinical point of view it is important to note that proton pump inhibitors inhibit H. pylori's urease [24]. This might contribute to the antibacterial effect of these drugs and can also cause false-negative urease results during therapy. The genes encoding the two subunits of urease, *ureA* and *ureB*, have been cloned [25,26].The enzyme urease is clearly beneficial to *H. pylori* but the ammonium ions that it produces may be injurious to the host (see below and Chapter 3).

Proton pump
H. pylori has an H^+/K^+ ATPase 'proton pump' of the P-type nor-mally found in parietal cells [27]. This is unusual in bacteria and probably acts to maintain the 1:1 000 000 proton gradient across the bacterial cell membrane, by 'baling out' any protons that get into the bacterium.

Motility
When viewed *in vivo* under the microscope or on video, *H. pylori* are actually highly motile, a point entirely missed by the familiar still photographs. In the stomach *H. pylori* use their spiral shape and flagellae to drill themselves to sites that are moderately acidic. The stomach is lined by a layer of mucus. The gastric epithelium secretes bicarbonate into the mucus layer at about 10% of the rate of acid secretion so that the pH on the surface of the epithelial cells is close to neutral. *H. pylori* bacteria colonize this zone, although by doing so they may increase the permeability of the mucus layer to back-diffusion of acid. *H. pylori* also prefers the antrum, where parietal cells are absent or scanty. However, when acid secretion is suppressed, the bacteria migrate into the corpus [28], perhaps attracted by the remaining acid secretion. This migration is clinically important because it leads to misleadingly negative antral biopsies during omeprazole therapy. For the same reason an improvement in antral gastritis during suppression of acid secretion may be accompanied by a worsening of gastritis in the gastric corpus [29].

The importance of motility was also demonstrated in the gnotobiotic piglets. Strains of *H. pylori* which were immobile because they lacked flagellae were less able to colonize these animals [30].

Coping with immune and inflammatory factors

An important feature of *H. pylori* is the ability to survive in the stomach despite the mucosal immune response. How it does this is poorly understood. However the mechanisms involved are important clinically because they will have to be overcome before immunization can succeed. Fortunately, studies in mice infected with *H. pylori* and *H. felis* show that immunity capable of preventing and even eradicating the infection can be produced by adding adjuvants such as cholera toxin to *Helicobacter* antigens [31,32].

Luminal location
The immune response of the gastrointestinal tract is only moderately successful against bacteria such as *H. pylori*, which remain in the lumen. This as illustrated by slow clearance of other pathogenic bacteria such as *Clostridium difficile*. The low pH in the stomach lumen may further impair the effect of IgA antibodies against *H. pylori*.

Shedding antigens
H. pylori sheds large amounts of antigens such as urease from its surface. Shed antigens may 'mop-up' IgA antibodies secreted into the lumen.

Feeble endotoxin
Bacterial endotoxins (lipopolysaccharides) are often highly potent activators of leucocytes, but the endotoxin of *H. pylori* is unusually feeble in this respect [33].

Catalase – versus H_2O_2
One way in which neutrophils attack bacteria is by releasing oxygen free radicals. *H. pylori* produces the enzyme catalase, which dissipates these by converting hydrogen peroxide to water and oxygen gas [34].

Heat-shock proteins
Heat-shock proteins act as chaperones for protein molecules, stabilizing and probably also repairing them under harsh

conditions. They are produced by all cells, and this includes *H. pylori* bacteria and the gastric epithelium [35]. They are so-called because their production is increased when cells are stressed by thermal, chemical or physical stress. This includes bacterial challenge of human tissues [36]. *H. pylori*'s heat-shock proteins may allow it to survive the harsh conditions in the stomach. However antibodies against bacterial heat-shock proteins might act as auto-antibodies by cross-reacting with the host's heat-shock proteins in the gastric mucosa [37].

Negative feedback
It is easy to envisage that *H.-pylori*-induced mucosal damage will increase delivery of bacterial antigens to the immune system and thus lead to even more inflammation and damage. The fact that inflammation and damage are limited suggests the existence of at least one negative-feedback loop. Perhaps damage leads to killing of bacteria by factors such as antibodies and leucocytes in exuded serum?

It is also possible that by confining itself (more or less) to the stomach *H. pylori* avoids delivering antigens to the Peyer's patches in the ileum where they would stimulate the immune system more strongly.

RESTRICTION TO THE GASTRIC MUCOSA

H. pylori is not only adapted to live in the stomach but is also only able to colonize gastric epithelium. This important feature of *H. pylori* might be due to the specific binding of *H. pylori* to gastric cells of the surface and foveolar type. About 20% of bacteria are attached in this way, sometimes through an adhesion pedestal [38]. Adhesion is through bacterial **adhesins**, which adhere to specific motifs on the cell surface. These include membrane-associated phospholipids such as phosphatidyl ethanolamine [39,40]. Another adhesin binds to the sialic acid sugar N-acetyl muraminyl lactose. [41,42]. It is particularly interesting that one adhesin appears to bind to the Lewis B blood group antigen, possibly more so if it is associated with blood group O rather than blood groups A or B [43]. Adhesion of *H. pylori* to specific blood group motifs may also explain why certain upper gastrointestinal diseases tend to occur in people with particular blood groups. Disease outcome also depends on whether the patient is a 'secretor' who secretes blood group substances into saliva and other bodily secretions, or a 'non-secretor' who does not. It is easy to imagine that adhesion might be less if bacteria are coated with Lewis B antigen secreted into the gastric lumen. Also, different strains of *H. pylori* have different adhesins. Therefore, whether adhesion occurs or not depends on both the bacteria and the host. Adhesion may restrict bacterial colonization to the stomach, but may also contribute to tissue damage. Adhesion may facilitate presentation of bacterial antigens to the immune system and increase exposure of the epithelium to bacterial toxins. Patients with the greatest adhesion tend to have more severe epithelial damage [44] (Chapter 3).

H. pylori also colonizes heterotopic or metaplastic gastric epithelium outside the stomach (Figure 1.3). This includes patches of metaplastic gastric epithelium in the duodenal bulb of patients with duodenal ulcers [45] and Barrett's epithelium in the oesophagus of patients with chronic acid reflux. About 50% of Barrett's oesophagi are colonized with *H. pylori*, and infection there appears to increase the frequency of oesophageal ulcers [46]. Ectopic gastric epithelium in Meckel's diverticula can also become colonized [47]. *H. pylori* has even been found on patches of ectopic gastric-type

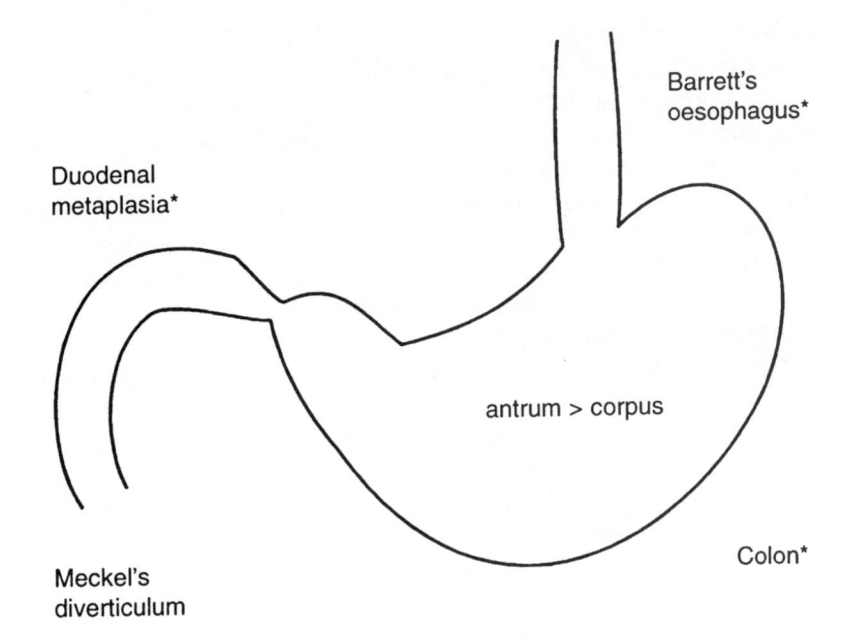

Figure 1.3 Sites of *H. pylori* infection reported in humans. *indicates sites of gastric metaplasia.

epithelium in the rectum [48]. These patches were inflamed, but the surrounding mucosa was not. The discovery of *H. pylori* in the rectum emphasizes that this bacterium does pass right through the gut and out in the faeces.

MULTIPLE STRAINS

There are many different strains of *H. pylori*. These can be distinguished by making fingerprints of bacterial proteins or DNA. This approach has been used to make some clinically important points: 're-infection' in 'the West' is usually actually due to re-growth of the same strain [25]. This is most probably because the infection was not really eradicated in the first place. It is also possible that the patient is truly re-infected, but from a close relative. Fingerprinting has shown that about a half of infected family members are infected with the same strain [49,50]. If this proves to be a common occurrence, should the whole family be treated?

Toxigenic strains

Vacuolating toxin and cagA
An important feature of *H. pylori* is that it can be divided into toxigenic and non-toxigenic strains. It was first noticed that some strains but not others produce a factor 'vacuolating toxin' which produces acid vacuoles in mammalian cells. Interestingly 67% of patients with ulcers had strains which produced this toxin, compared with only 30% of patients without ulcers. Vacuolating toxin is a 87 kDa protein encoded by the gene *vacA* [51]. Molecular studies indicate that this gene comes in one of two different forms. Strains which produce vacuolating toxin have *1vacA*, while strains which do not produce the toxin possess the *2vacA* version of the gene [52]. Therefore, one might expect serological studies to show antibodies to vacuolating toxin more often in ulcer patients. However no such difference has been found. This might be because the vacuolating toxin is not very antigenic, or because the product of *2vacA* has the same epitopes. Instead, ulcer patients more often have antibodies to the 120–128 kDa product of gene *cagA* [53]. Differences in the size of the protein are due to variability in the number of repeating sequences in the gene. In one such study mucosal IgA antibodies to this protein were present in 100% of ulcer patients compared with about 70% of controls [54]. This gene is present in all strains which

have *1vacA* and therefore produce the vacuolating toxin. However it is only present in about a third of strains which have gene *2vacA* and are therefore non-toxigenic (Figure 1.4). The idea that *cagA* and *vacA* are important in pathogenesis is attractive, but it should be remembered that Western blotting and ELISAs do not measure these products but the antibodies to them. Therefore some results may reflect the strength of the host's immune response and the number of bacteria as well as the nature of the strain. Vacuolating toxin has been identified in human faeces [55], raising the interesting possibility that *H. pylori* might cause disease in the lower gut.

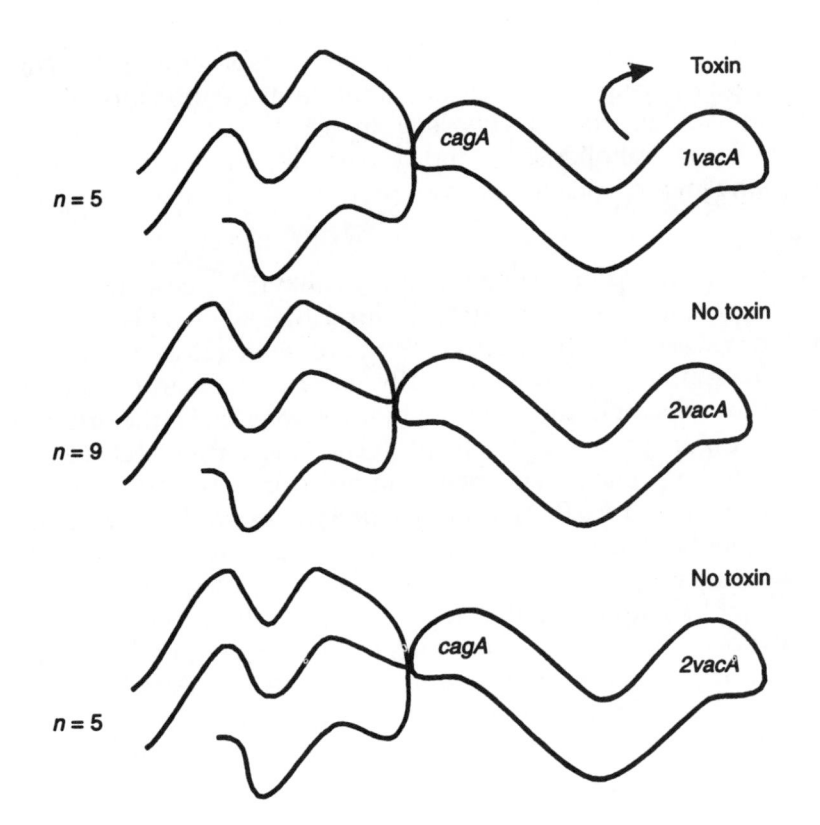

Figure 1.4 Different strains of *H. pylori*, as described by Atherton *et al.* (*Source*: redrawn from reference 52, with permission.)

Other aggressive factors produced by *H. pylori*

The attraction and activation of leucocytes
Apart from its feeble endotoxin [56], *H. pylori* releases several factors which attract and activate leucocytes. These include a 10.5 kDa molecule reported from Michigan [57], a < 3 kDa molecule described from Los Angeles [58] and a molecule resembling the N-formyl peptide f-Met-Leu-Phe produced by other bacteria, which has been reported from New Zealand [59]. A water extract of *H. pylori* promoted the adherence of CD molecules on neutrophils to ICAM-1 on epithelial cells; a process that precedes their migration into tissue fluid [60]. One study suggests that strains associated with peptic ulcers have more potent neutrophil-activating activity [61].

Phospholipase
H. pylori possesses the lipolytic enzyme phospholipase A_2. This digests phospholipids, which are important components of cell membranes. One product is lysolecithin, which is cytotoxic. Concentrations of phospholipase A_2 and lysolecithin are both elevated in the gastric juice of infected persons [62].

Ammonium ions
Ammonium ions produced by *H. pylori*'s enzyme urease may damage the gastric mucosa. Megraud found that wild-type *H. pylori* produce vacuoles in HEp2 cells while a urease-negative mutant did not [63]. Ammonium ions generally expand the acidic vacuoles present in cells, and ammonium chloride potentiates the effect of vacuolating toxin on HeLa cells [64]. The long-term effects of ammonia on the stomach have been examined in rats. Replacing the drinking water with 0.01% ammonia for 8 weeks produced atrophic changes in the gastric antrum and increased proliferation throughout the stomach [65]. This treatment also promoted gastric carcinogenesis [66]. Gastric juice ammonium concentrations correlate with the severity of gastritis in man [67], but findings in patients with uraemia argue against ammonia as an important cause of gastritis: uninfected patients with renal failure had much less gastritis than infected controls, even though both groups had similar intragastric ammonium levels [68].

HELICOBACTERS IN ANIMALS

Why mention the helicobacters of animals in a 'clinician's guide'? Helicobacters in animals are clinically important because they occasionally infect humans. Studies of infected animals are useful in the development of new ways to prevent and treat human *H. pylori* infection, as well as in the exploration of pathogenic mechanisms. Helicobacters from each animal species are often quite specific for that animal. They are all regarded as helicobacters because of similarities in the sequence of the gene that encodes 16S rRNA, a component of the bacterial ribosome [15]. Lee is the international authority in this area and has recently written an excellent review [69].

The bacteria

Helicobacter mustelae
This is a small curved rod found in the stomach of ferrets [70].

Helicobacter felis
The stomachs of cats and dogs often contain huge numbers of at least three different helicobacters. *H. felis* is more tightly coiled than *H. pylori* and has prominent periplasmic fibrils [71]. It seems equally at home in dogs and cats. There have been two reports of humans infected with *H. felis*. In both cases there was an acute neutrophilic gastritis [72,73].

'Helicobacter heilmanni' ('*Gastrospirillum hominis*'), etc.
The predominant spiral bacterium in cats and dogs is not *H. felis* but a tightly coiled bacterium without periplasmic fibrils. This is the most common type of helicobacter in the animal kingdom. Interest was heightened when Dent observed a bacterium with this appearance in biopsies from three out of 1300 patients with histological gastritis [74]. The infection was thought to have come from the patients' pets [75] and tentatively named *Gastrospirillum hominis*. This bacterium is now thought to cause about 1% of human gastritis. It has not been cultured *in vitro* but grows readily in the mouse stomach [76]. Analysis of the 16S ribosomal RNA gene indicates that it belongs to the genus *Helicobacter* and the name *H. heilmanni* has been tentatively assigned to a human isolate [77]. The important clinical point is that similar organisms are present in the stomachs of many animals, so these will occasionally turn up in patients' stomachs.

Helicobacter acinonyx
The most exotic helicobacter found so far was isolated from a colony of cheetahs in Ohio. These animals became seriously ill with chronic

vomiting. Histology showed a severe gastritis and tightly spiralled bacteria which looked like '*H. heilmanni*' and could not be cultured. However it was possible to culture a different bacterium, which resembled *H. pylori* and was named *Helicobacter acinonyx* [78].

Non-gastric helicobacters
Bacteria are defined as helicobacters partly by analysis of sequences in their 16S ribosomal RNA gene. Based on this, some bacteria have been discovered or re-classified as helicobacters, even though they do not produce urease or colonize the stomach. These include *H. cinaedi*, *H. fennelliae* and *H. canis*, and are mentioned to complete the picture.

Natural and experimental infection in animals

Primates
Many species of primates are colonized with '*H. heilmanni*' [79]. In addition, bacteria almost identical to *H. pylori* have been found in a range of primates. These may have been transmitted to the animals by their keepers. It would be interesting to know whether primates in the wild are infected. *H. pylori* produces gastritis in primates in the same way that it does in humans.

Pigs and piglets
H. pylori will colonize gnotobiotic piglets (i.e. animals with a defined bacterial flora), in which it produces a gastritis similar to that seen in children, with prominent mononuclear cell infiltrate and lymphoid follicles [80]. This model has been used to show that strains which lack urease or motility do not colonize the stomach normally [22,30].

Ferrets
Ferrets infected with *H. mustelae* are in many ways the best model of human disease because the animals develop atrophy and occasionally even develop ulcers at the pylorus or duodenum [79]. A high percentage of bacteria adhere to the gastric epithelium in this model [79]. Ferrets have proved useful in trials of antimicrobial therapy [81].

Dogs and cats
In both species *H. felis* produces a gastritis with marked lymphoid follicles [82]. Both species can also be infected with *H. pylori*. Indeed

domestic cats purchased from one out of four vendors in the USA were found to be infected with the human bacteria [83].

Mice
Mice do not have natural gastric *Helicobacter* but are readily colonized with *H. felis* and this is the most popular model for research into immunization [32]. The histological response varies from strain to strain, emphasizing the importance of host factors. In some instances atrophic gastritis and even early dysplasia are seen [84], but mice infected with *H. felis* do not develop ulcers.

CONCLUSIONS

Helicobacter pylori is uniquely adapted to the gastric milieu. It has mechanisms to deal with gastric acid and local immune and inflammatory factors. Some strains of *H. pylori* are more likely to cause disease than others. Animals are frequently infected with their own helicobacters and these occasionally infect the human stomach. The discovery of these bacteria is both a remarkable story and a major medical advance.

REFERENCES

1. Black JW, Duncan WA, Durant CJ *et al*. Definition and antagonism of histamine H_2-receptors. *Nature* 1972; **236**: 385–390.
2. Elcenved G, Carlsson E, Cederberg C *et al*. Studies with H168/68, a novel gastric acid secretion inhibitor (abstract). *Gut* 1981; **22**: A877.
3. Bottcher G. *Dorpater Med Z* 1874; **5**: 148.
4. Salomon H. Ueber das Spirillum des Saugetiermagens und sein Verhalten zu den Belegzellen. *Zentralbl Bakteriol* 1896; **19**: 433–442.
5. Krienitz W. Ueber das Auftreten von Spirochaetne verschiegener Form im Magen-inhalt bei Carcinoma ventriculi. *Dtsch Med Wochenschr* 1906; **32**: 872.
6. Palmer ED. Investigation of the gastric mucosa spirochaetes of the human. *Gastroenterology* 1954; **27**: 218–220.
7. Luck JM, Seth TN. Gastric urease. *Biochem J* 1924; **18**: 1227–1231.
8. Langenberg M, Tytgat GN, Schipper MEI *et al*. *Campylobacter*-like organisms in the stomach of patients and healthy individuals (letter). *Lancet* 1984; **i**: 1348–1349.

9. Steer HW. Ultrastructure of cell migration through the gastric epithelium and its relationship to bacteria. *J Clin Pathol* 1975; **28**: 639–646.
10. Fung WP, Papadimitriou JM, Matz LR. Endoscopic, histological and ultrastructural correlations in chronic gastritis. *Am J Gastroenterol* 1979; **71**: 269–279.
11. Warren JR. Unidentified curved bacilli on gastric epithelium in active chronic gastritis (letter). *Lancet* 1983; **i**: 1273.
12. Marshall BJ, Warren JR. Unidentified curved bacilli in the stomach of patients with gastritis and peptic ulceration. *Lancet* 1984; **i**: 1311–1315.
13. Rollason TP, Stone J, Rhodes JM. Spiral organisms in endoscopic biopsies of the human stomach. *J Clin Pathol* 1984; **37**: 23–26.
14. Steer HW. Surface morphology of the gastroduodenal mucosa in duodenal ulceration. *Gut* 1984; **25**: 1203–1210.
15. Goodwin CS, Armstrong JA, Chilvers T *et al.* Transfer of *Campylobacter pylori* and *Campylobacter mustelae* to *Helicobacter* gen. nov. and *Helicobacter pylori* comb. nov. and *Helicobacter mustelae* comb. nov., respectively. *Int J Syst Bacteriol* 1989; **39**: 397–405.
16. Graham DY, Alpert LC, Smith JL, Yoshimura HH. Iatrogenic *Campylobacter pylori* infection is a cause of epidemic achlorhydria. *Am J Gastroenterol* 1988; **83**: 974–980.
17. Cave DR, Vargas M. Effect of a *Campylobacter pylori* protein on acid secretion by parietal cells. *Lancet* 1989; **ii**: 187–189.
18. Tache Y, Saperas E. Potent inhibition of gastric acid secretion and ulcer formation by centrally and peripherally administered interleukin-1. *Ann N Y Acad Sci* 1992; **664**: 353–368.
19. Berglund H, Chang HC. Transitory character of the achlorhydria during fever demonstrated by the histamine test. *Proc R Soc Exp Biol Med* 1929; **26**: 422–423.
20. Hu LT, Mobley HL. Expression of catalytically active recombinant *Helicobacter pylori* urease at wild-type levels in *Escherichia coli*. *Infect Immun* 1993; **61**: 2563–2569.
21. Marshall BJ, Barrett LJ, Prakash C *et al.* Urea protects *Helicobacter* (*Campylobacter*) *pylori* from the bactericidal effect of acid. *Gastroenterology* 1990; **99**: 697–702.
22. Eaton KA, Brooks CL, Morgan DR, Krakowka S. Essential role of urease in pathogenesis of gastritis induced by *Helicobacter pylori* in gnotobiotic piglets. *Infect Immun* 1991; **59**: 2470–2475.
23. Butcher GP, Ryder SD, Hughes SJ *et al.* Use of an ammonia

electrode for rapid quantification of *Helicobacter pylori* urease: its use in the endoscopy room and in the assessment of urease inhibition by bismuth subsalicylate. *Digestion* 1992; **53**: 142–148.

24. Nagata K, Satoh H, Iwahi T *et al.* Potent inhibitory action of the gastric proton pump inhibitor lansoprazole against urease activity of *Helicobacter pylori*: unique action selective for *H. pylori* cells. *Antimicrob Agents Chemother* 1993; **37**: 769–774.

25. Clayton CL, Kleanthous H, Morgan DD, Puckey L, Tabaqchali S. Rapid fingerprinting of *Helicobacter pylori* by polymerase chain reaction and restriction fragment length polymorphism analysis. *J Clin Microbiol* 1993; **31**: 1420–1425.

26. Labigne A, Cussac V, Courcoux P. Shuttle cloning and nucleotide sequences of *Helicobacter pylori* genes responsible for urease activity. *J Bacteriol* 1991; **173**: 1920–1931.

27. Mauch F, Bode G, Malfertheiner P. Identification and characterization of an ATPase system of *Helicobacter pylori* and the effect of proton pump inhibitors (letter). *Am J Gastroenterol* 1993; **88**: 1801–1802.

28. Logan RPH, Walker MM, Misiewicz JJ *et al.* Changes in the intragastric distribution of *Helicobacter pylori* during treatment with omeprazole. *Gut* 1995; **36**: 12–16.

29. Unge P, Gad A, Gnarpe H, Olsson J. Does omeprazole improve antimicrobial therapy directed towards gastric *Campylobacter pylori* in patients with antral gastritis? A pilot study. *Scand J Gastroenterol* 1989; **24**(suppl 167): 49–54.

30. Eaton KA, Morgan DR, Krakowka S. Motility as a factor in the colonisation of gnotobiotic piglets by *Helicobacter pylori*. *J Med Microbiol* 1992; **37**: 123–127.

31. Chen M, Lee A, Hazell S. Immunisation against gastric helicobacter infection in a mouse/*Helicobacter felis* model (letter). *Lancet* 1992; **339**: 1120–1121.

32. Doidge C, Crust I, Lee A *et al.* Therapeutic immunisation against *Helicobacter* infection (letter). *Lancet* 1994; **343**: 914–915.

33. Nielsen H, Birkholz S, Andersen LP, Moran AP. Neutrophil activation by *Helicobacter pylori* lipopolysaccharides. *J Infect Dis* 1994; **170**: 135–139.

34. Hazell SL, Evans DJ Jr, Graham DY. *Helicobacter pylori* catalase. *J Gen Microbiol* 1991; **137**: 57–61.

35. Dunn BE, Roop RM, Sung CC *et al.* Identification and purification of a cpn60 heat shock protein homolog from *Helicobacter pylori*. *Infect Immun* 1992; **60**: 1946–1951.

36. Kaufmann SH, Schoel B, van Embden JD *et al.* Heat-shock protein 60: implications for pathogenesis of and protection against bacterial infections. *Immunol Rev* 1991; **121**: 67–90.
37. Negrini R, Lisato L, Zanella I *et al. Helicobacter pylori* infection induces antibodies cross–reacting with human gastric mucosa. *Gastroenterology* 1991; **101**: 437–445.
38. Narikawa S, Imai N, Sakama S *et al.* Evaluation of agar media for growth of *Campylobacter pylori. Rinsho Byori* 1990; **38**: 104–106.
39. Gold BD, Huesca M, Sherman PM, Lingwood CA. *Helicobacter mustelae* and *Helicobacter pylori* bind to common lipid receptors in vitro. *Infect Immun* 1993; **61**: 2632–2638.
40. Lingwood CA, Wasfy G, Han H, Huesca M. Receptor affinity purification of a lipid-binding adhesin from *Helicobacter pylori. Infect Immun* 1993; **61**: 2474–2478.
41. Huang J, Keeling PW, Smyth CJ. Identification of erythrocyte-binding antigens in *Helicobacter pylori. J Gen Microbiol* 1992; **138**: 1503–1513.
42. Evans DG, Karjalainen TK, Evans DJ Jr *et al.* Cloning, nucleotide sequence, and expression of a gene encoding an adhesin subunit protein of *Helicobacter pylori. J Bacteriol* 1993; **175**: 674–683.
43. Boren T, Falk P, Roth KA *et al.* Attachment of *Helicobacter pylori* to human gastric epithelium mediated by blood group antigens. *Science* 1993; **262**: 1892–1895.
44. Hessey SJ, Spencer J, Wyatt JI *et al.* Bacterial adhesion and disease activity in *Helicobacter* associated chronic gastritis. *Gut* 1990; **31**: 134–138.
45. Wyatt JI, Rathbone BJ, Sobala GM *et al.* Gastric epithelium in the duodenum: its association with *Helicobacter pylori* and inflammation. *J Clin Pathol* 1990; **43**: 981–986.
46. Loffeld RJ, Ten Tije BJ, Arends JW. Prevalence and significance of *Helicobacter pylori* in patients with Barrett's esophagus. *Am J Gastroenterol* 1992; **87**: 1598–1600.
47. De Cothi GA, Newbold KM, O'Connor HJ. *Campylobacter*-like organisms and heterotopic gastric mucosa in Meckel's diverticula. *J Clin Pathol* 1989; **42**: 132–134.
48. Dye KR, Marshall BJ, Frierson HF Jr *et al. Campylobacter pylori* colonizing heterotopic gastric tissue in the rectum. *Am J Clin Pathol* 1990; **93**: 144–147.
49. Nwokolo CU, Bickley J, Attard AR *et al.* Evidence of clonal variants of *Helicobacter pylori* in three generations of a duodenal ulcer disease family. *Gut* 1992; **33**: 1323–1327.

50. Bamford KB, Bickley J, Collins JS *et al. Helicobacter pylori*: comparison of DNA fingerprints provides evidence for intrafamilial infection. *Gut* 1993; **34**: 1348–1350.
51. Cover TL, Blaser MJ. Purification and characterization of the vacuolating toxin from *Helicobacter pylori. J Biol Chem* 1992; **267**: 10570–10575.
52. Atherton JC, Cover TL, Peek RM, Blaser MJ. Subtyping of *Helicobacter pylori* strains into two groups by polymerase chain reaction amplification of the *vacA* gene and correlation of these groups with CagA status (abstract). *Am J Gastroenterol* 1994; **89**: 1291.
53. Tummuru MK, Cover TL, Blaser MJ. Cloning and expression of a high-molecular-mass major antigen of *Helicobacter pylori*: evidence of linkage to cytotoxin production. *Infect Immun* 1993; **61**: 1799–1809.
54. Crabtree JE, Taylor JD, Wyatt JI *et al.* Mucosal IgA recognition of *Helicobacter pylori* 120 kDa protein, peptic ulceration, and gastric pathology. *Lancet* 1991; **338**: 332–335.
55. Luzzi I, Pezzella C, Caprioli A *et al.* Detection of vacuolating toxin of *Helicobacter pylori* in human faeces (letter). *Lancet* 1993; **341**: 1348.
56. Rautelin H, Blomberg B, Fredlund H *et al.* Incidence of *Helicobacter pylori* strains activating neutrophils in patients with peptic ulcer disease. *Gut* 1993; **34**: 599–603.
57. Kozol R, McCurdy B, Czanko R. A neutrophil chemotactic factor present in *H. pylori* but absent in *H. mustelae. Dig Dis Sci* 1993; **38**: 137–141.
58. Craig PM, Territo MC, Karnes WE, Walsh JH. *Helicobacter pylori* secretes a chemotactic factor for monocytes and neutrophils. *Gut* 1992; **33**: 1020–1023.
59. Mooney C, Keenan J, Munster D *et al.* Neutrophil activation by *Helicobacter pylori. Gut* 1991; **32**: 853–857.
60. Yoshida N, Granger DN, Evans DJ Jr *et al.* Mechanisms involved in *Helicobacter pylori*-induced inflammation. *Gastroenterology* 1993; **105**: 1431–1440.
61. Muotiala A, Helander IM, Pyhala L *et al.* Low biological activity of *Helicobacter pylori* lipopolysaccharide. *Infect Immun* 1992; **60**: 1714–1716.
62. Langton SR, Cesareo SD. *Helicobacter pylori* associated phospholipase A_2 activity: a factor in peptic ulcer production? *J Clin Pathol* 1992; **45**: 221–224.
63. Megraud F, Neman Simha V, Brugmann D. Further evidence of

the toxic effect of ammonia produced by *Helicobacter pylori* urease on human epithelial cells. *Infect Immun* 1992; **60**: 1858–1863.

64. Cover TL, Vaughn SG, Cao P, Blaser MJ. Potentiation of *Helicobacter pylori* vacuolating toxin activity by nicotine and other weak bases. *J Infect Dis* 1992; **166**: 1073–1078.

65. Tsujii M, Kawano S, Tsuji S *et al.* Cell kinetics of mucosal atrophy in rat stomach induced by long-term administration of ammonia. *Gastroenterology* 1993; **104**: 796–801.

66. Tsujii M, Kawano S, Tsuji S *et al.* Ammonia: a possible promotor in *Helicobacter pylori*-related gastric carcinogenesis. *Cancer Lett* 1992; **65**: 15–18.

67. Triebling AT, Korsten MA, Dlugosz JW *et al.* Severity of *Helicobacter*-induced gastric injury correlates with gastric juice ammonia. *Dig Dis Sci* 1991; **36**: 1089–1096.

68. El Nujumi AM, Rowe PA, Dahill S *et al.* Role of ammonia in the pathogenesis of the gastritis, hypergastrinaemia, and hyperpepsinogenaemia I caused by *Helicobacter pylori* infection. *Gut* 1992; **33**: 1612–1616.

69. Lee A. Animal models and vaccine development. In: Calam J, ed. *Baillière's Clinical Gastroenterology: Helicobacter pylori*. London: Baillière Tindall, 1995: **9**: 615–632.

70. Fox JG, Edrise BM, Cabot EB *et al. Campylobacter*-like organisms isolated from gastric mucosa of ferrets. *Am J Vet Res* 1986; **47**: 236–239.

71. Lee A, Hazell SL, O'Rourke J, Kouprach S. Isolation of a spiral-shaped bacterium from the cat stomach. *Infect Immun* 1988; **56**: 2843–2850.

72. Wegmann W, Aschwanden M, Schaub N *et al.* [Gastritis associated with *Gastrospirillum hominis* – a zoonosis?]. *Schweiz Med Wochenschr* 1991; **121**: 245–254.

73. Lavelle J, Conklin F, Mitros S, Landas S. Transmission of 'Gastrospirillum hominis' from cat to man. *Gastroenterology* 1992; **102**: A651.

74. Dent JC, McNulty CA, Uff JC *et al.* Spiral organisms in the gastric antrum (letter). *Lancet* 1987; **ii**: 96.

75. Lee A, Dent J, Hazell S, McNulty C. Origin of spiral organisms in human gastric antrum (letter). *Lancet* 1988; **i**: 300–301.

76. Dick E, Lee A, Watson G, O'Rourke J. Use of the mouse for the isolation and investigation of stomach-associated, spiral-helical shaped bacteria from man and other animals. *J Med Microbiol* 1989; **29**: 55–62.

77. Kuipers EJ, Pena AS, Van Kamp G *et al.* Seroconversion for *Helicobacter pylori. Lancet* 1993; **342**: 328–331.
78. Eaton KA, Radin MJ, Kramer L *et al.* Gastric spiral bacilli in captive cheetahs. *Scand J Gastroenterol Suppl* 1991; **181**: 38–42.
79. Fox JG, Lee A. Gastric *Helicobacter* infection in animals: natural and experimental infections. In: Goodwin CS, Worsley BW, eds. *Helicobacter pylori: biology and clincal practice.* Boca Raton, FL: CRC Press, 1993: 407–430.
80. Bertram TA, Murray PD, Morgan DR *et al.* Gastritis associated with infection by *Helicobacter pylori* in humans: geographical differences. *Scand J Gastroenterol Suppl* 1991; **181**: 1–8.
81. McColm AA, Bagshaw JA, O'Malley CF. Development of a ^{14}C-urea breath test in ferrets colonised with *Helicobacter mustelae*: effects of treatment with bismuth, antibiotics, and urease inhibitors. *Gut* 1993; **34**: 181–186.
82. Henry GA, Long PH, Burns JL, Charbonneau DL. Gastric spirillosis in beagles. *Am J Vet Res* 1987; **48**: 831–836.
83. Handt LK, Fox JG, Dewhirst FE *et al. Helicobacter pylori* isolated from the domestic cat: public health implications. *Infect Immun* 1994; **62**: 2367–2374.
84. Lee A, Chen M, Coltro N *et al.* Long term infection of the gastric mucosa with Helicobacter species does induce atrophic gastritis in an animal model of *Helicobacter pylori* infection. *Int J Med Microbiol Virol Parasitol Infect Dis* 1993; **280**: 38–50.

2

Epidemiology, spread and re-infection

INTRODUCTION

If we are going to control *H. pylori* infection we first need to know who is infected and how they contracted the infection. Feldman has recently written an excellent review of this topic [1]. Studies in this area pose several problems. The groups of people being compared must be carefully matched. For instance, the question of whether farm animals are an important source of infection was confused by studies comparing the prevalence of infection in abattoir workers with the prevalence in controls who were not matched for other factors that affect transmission of the bacterium. The test used to detect infection must also be accurate. For example, it is not clear whether abattoir workers have false-positive results due to exposure to related bacteria in the animals that they slaughter. The urea breath test is more accurate than serology for the diagnosis of *H. pylori* but more cumbersome to perform. A further problem is that transmission in the West is a rare event and difficult to study directly. Despite all these difficulties knowledge is expanding rapidly and we already know much. Hopefully the information that is being gathered will indicate how infection, re-infection and the associated diseases can be prevented.

WHO IS INFECTED?

Age and the cohort effect

The prevalence of *H. pylori* infection increases with age. In the Western world the percentage of the population that is infected rises gradually from infancy to an age of about 60 years. Positive serology is uncommon in children, but present in about 20% of persons under the age of 40 years, and about 50% of those over the age of 60 years (Figure 2.1) [2,3]. The prevalence in the elderly may be an underestimate because serology often gives false-negative results in older people. This may be because gastric atrophy diminishes the number of organisms present [4].

A simple explanation for the rates of infection in the Western world might be that about 1% of the population acquire the infection each year. However this is not the whole story because careful studies have shown that the rate of acquisition is only 0.3–0.5% per patient year in Western adults [5,6]. The answer to this riddle lies in the observation that the prevalence of *H. pylori* infection is actually falling quite rapidly in the West [7]. At any given age the percentage of people who are infected is now lower than it was 20 years ago

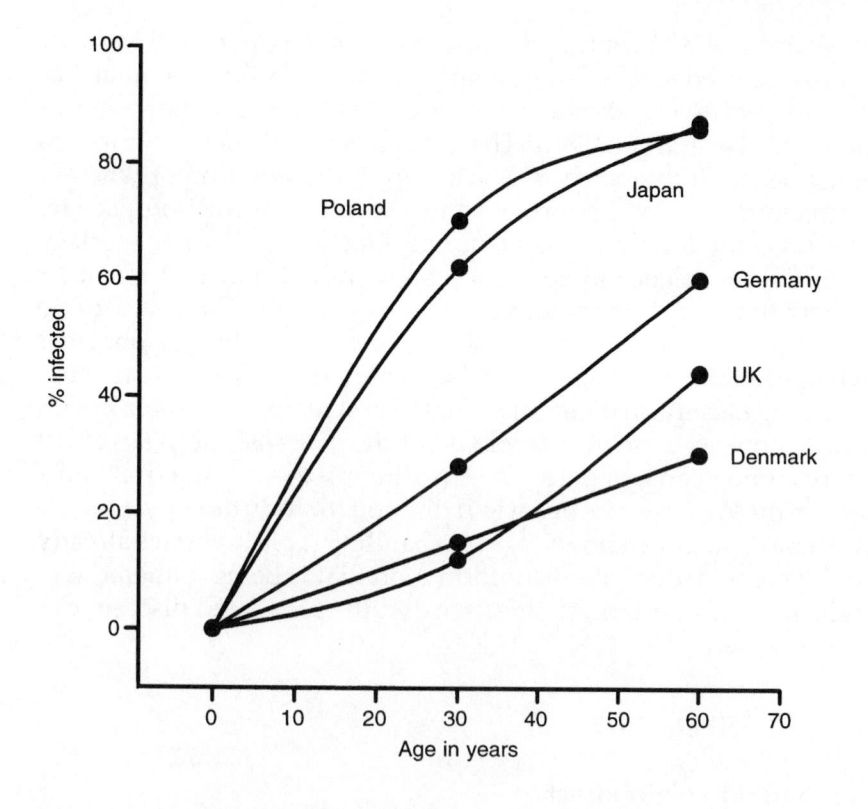

Figure 2.1 The prevalence of *H. pylori* at different ages in different countries. (*Source*: from data in reference 3.)

(Figure 2.2). Parsonnet found that the prevalence of *H. pylori* in epidemiologists over the age of 30 years has fallen from 43% in 1969–1974 to 21% in recent years [5]. Therefore the higher prevalence of the infection in elderly people is partly due to a 'cohort effect' [7]. In other words the people who are old now are have a higher prevalence of infection because they were alive at a time when *H. pylori* was considerably more prevalent than it is now. It seems likely that they mostly acquired *H. pylori* infection in childhood. Conditions then were more like they are now in developing countries (see below).

It is generally thought that the recent fall in the prevalence of *H. pylori* in Western countries is due to improvements in sanitation

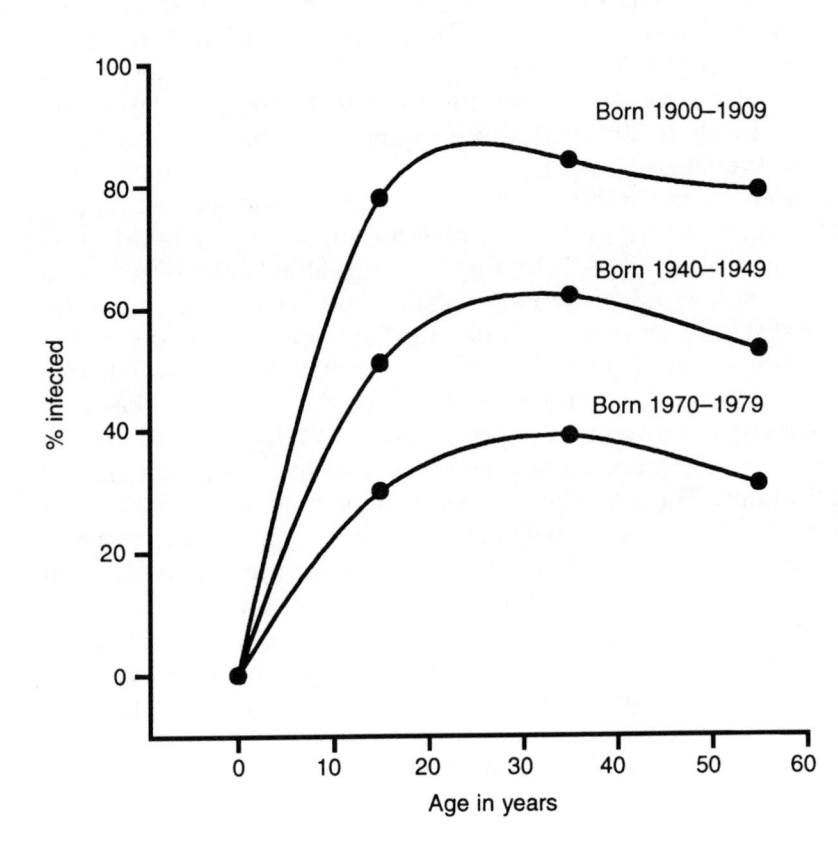

Figure 2.2 The prevalence of *H. pylori* at different ages in Western countries now and in the past; a computer model including extrapolation into the future. (*Source*: from data in reference 7.)

and living conditions. However a relative freedom from major wars involving Western troops since 1948 might also have contributed. It is easy to imagine that soldiers might catch the infection from each other through close contact and poor sanitation in a battle zone. Consistent with this, 7% of American servicemen acquired the infection during a period of only 6 months in the Gulf War [8]. Soldiers returning from wars may then spread *H. pylori* among family and friends.

Geographical differences

The pattern of *H. pylori* infection in developing countries is quite different from the pattern seen in the West [9]. Of course there are differences between and within these countries [10] but studies in Latin America [10,11], India [12], Africa, China and South-east Asia [9] show that in many communities most of the population are infected by their 20th birthday (Figure 2.2). This is presumably because transmission of *H. pylori* is increased by inadequate living conditions, overcrowding and suboptimal hygiene and sanitation.

The same factors probably cause the much higher re-infection rates that are seen in developing countries after patients have had the infection eradicated. For instance 20% of patients were re-infected within 18 months of having their infection eradicated in Brazil [13]. Eradication was not diagnosed by the urea breath test so it is possible that the treatment suppressed the infection rather than eradicating it. However, if re-infection rates really are much higher in these environments, as seems likely, this has important clinical implications. There is clearly less to be gained from eradicating *H. pylori* if the patient will soon be re-infected. Interestingly, members of ethnic groups from developing countries have elevated infection rates even if they are born in the West, and this is not entirely explained by differences in socioeconomic status [2,11]. Second-generation immigrants might have greater exposure to infection from infected parents or while visiting relatives abroad. In addition, their family practices, such as dipping chopsticks into a communal bowl (see below) might be more likely to spread the infection than normal Western habits.

Education, income and living conditions

One universal finding has been that this infection is more prevalent in groups with inferior education and lower incomes. For example infection rates in the Eurogast study were 34% in adults with higher education, 47% in those with secondary education and 62% in people who only received primary education [3]. Nobody has suggested (yet) that *H. pylori* can be eradicated by periods of study. Of course education is actually an indirect index of the hygiene facilities and practices that determine whether *H. pylori* is transmitted or not. Wealth is another index of the same thing. Poorer people acquire *H. pylori* infection at a younger age and their cumulative infection rate is also higher. For example infection rates in 6–11-year-olds in America were 10% in high-income families compared with 50% in poor families [14]. The role of living conditions during childhood was highlighted in a study in the United Kingdom. Whether adults are infected or not depends more on the conditions in their childhood home than on their current socioeconomic status. People who shared a bed as children were twice as likely to be infected with *H. pylori* as people who did not, even after correcting for their age and income at the time of testing [15]. Absence of hot water in the childhood home increased the risk in one study [16] but not in another [15].

Infection within the family and at school

H. pylori is spread largely by person-to-person contact. Therefore one would expect transmission to occur most often in the home. Clustering of the infection within families is evidence for this. In a study in Toronto 81% of the siblings of infected children were infected with *H. pylori* compared with only 13% of the siblings of uninfected children. Similarly 83% of parents of infected children were infected compared with only 27% of parents of uninfected children [17] (Figure 2.3). Studies of married couples also indicate the importance of children as vectors for *H. pylori* infection in Western countries. Family studies have shown that there is concordance between infection between the parents. However there was no concordance between infection in childless couples attending an infertility clinic [18]. This finding also suggests that *H. pylori* is not transmitted by sexual intercourse which the couples hoping to become parents were presumably performing to maximum capacity! There is also evidence that *H. pylori* is transmitted between children at school. Infection rates in schoolchildren in Edinburgh depended on the predominant socioeconomic group in the school that they attended, even after correcting for their parents' socioeconomic status. The idea that *H. pylori* may be acquired from inside

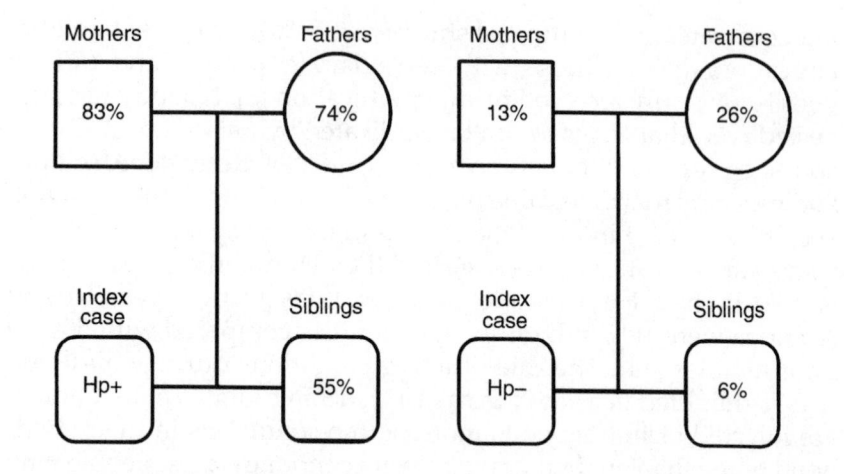

Figure 2.3 The prevalence of *H. pylori* in members of families in Toronto depending on whether one of the children was infected. (*Source*: from data in reference 17.)

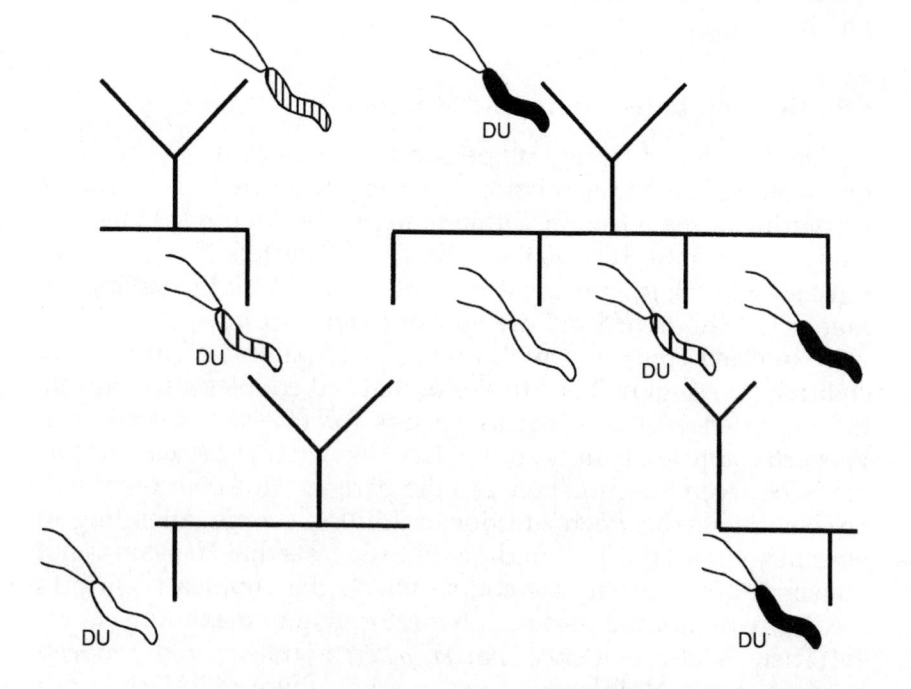

Figure 2.4 The presence of the same and different strains of *H. pylori* in three generations. The different strains are indicated by different shading. (*Source*: from reference 19, with permission.)

or outside the family is supported by DNA fingerprinting of strains in three generations of the same family (Figure 2.4). One member of each generation had the same strain, but other members of the same family were infected with other strains [19].

Occupation

Gastroenterologists are infected with *H. pylori* more often than members of other medical specialities [20]. This might be an exception to the general rule that wealthy Westerners are not infected. We probably acquired the infection while doing gastroscopies in the early days when it was quite usual to have gastric juice bubbling from the biopsy port a few centimetres from one's face. We were not particularly careful to protect ourselves because we thought that gastric juice was sterilized by its low pH. Hopefully measures introduced to prevent the spread of hepatitis virus and HIV have also decreased the transmission of *H. pylori* in the endoscopy room. It is often stated that this is due to endoscopists not wearing gloves in the early days of endoscopy, but the lack of a face-mask may be more relevant. Submariners are another occupational group with a high prevalence of *H. pylori* infection. It is not clear why they are infected more often than other servicemen [21]. One of the more repeatable theories is that high outside pressures lead to faeces passing in the wrong direction when the WC is flushed. The evidence that abattoir workers are infected more often than controls is discussed below.

Breast feeding

Mothers who are infected with *H. pylori* secrete IgA antibodies to the bacteria in their milk. Exposure of infants to *H. pylori* is extremely high in the Gambia. A study in that country showed that infants whose mothers had high titres of anti-*H. pylori* IgA in their milk were less likely to acquire the infection during suckling than the infants of mothers with low titres of these antibodies [22].

HOW DO INFECTION AND RE-INFECTION OCCUR?

Spread by animals or foods

Several studies have asked whether there is an important animal reservoir of *H. pylori* bacteria. The general conclusion has been that there is not. However the recent discovery that *H. pylori* is present in the stomachs of domestic cats raises the possibility that this might be a significant reservoir [23]. Researchers in the USA purchased domestic cats from four vendors. All of 22 cats bought from one vendor had *H. pylori*-like bacteria visible on gastric histology. The bacterium was successfully cultured from 75% of these and closely resembled *H. pylori* on detailed biochemical analysis. There is already evidence that helicobacters can be acquired from domestic animals: a 12-year-old Australian girl caught '*H. heilmanni*' (*Gastrospirillum hominis*) infection from her dog [24]. However a study in England showed that the prevalence of *H. pylori* infection did not depend on whether the family had pet animals or not [15].

Early evidence for significant transmission of helicobacters from animals to man came from studies in abattoir workers. These employees were found to have circulating antibodies to *H. pylori* more often than controls [25–27]. Unfortunately these results are generally rejected on the basis that the abattoir workers and controls were not matched for socioeconomic status. However another study found that people who had only worked at the abattoir for 1–2 years had higher titres of antibody against *H. pylori* than carefully matched controls [28]. Therefore it remains possible that abattoir workers do acquire *H. pylori* infection from animals that they kill. However it is also necessary to consider that exposure to animals' bacteria might produce antibodies that cross-react with antigens in the serological test for *H. pylori*. These results from abattoirs raised the possibility that *H. pylori* might enter the home environment through contaminated raw meat. It was shown that this bacterium can survive in chilled food for several days [29]. However neither vegetarians [30,31] nor other groups who do not eat either pork or beef [9] had *H. pylori* infection any less often than omnivorous controls.

Spread by water

In Western countries drinking water flows into the home through one pipe and excrement passes out through a completely separate one. Sadly this is not always the case in developing countries, where drinking water plays an important role in faecal–oral transmission of diseases. There is good evidence that *H. pylori* is transmitted via water in some parts of the world. It has been shown that *H. pylori* can survive for up to 3 days in water [32–34]. It seems that *H. pylori* is often spread by water in some regions of South America. This was shown in part of Peru where the domestic water comes either from the municipal supply or from community wells. Some people have to obtain municipal water from taps in the street while others have it piped into their homes. The prevalence of *H. pylori* infection in children in this area depended more on the source of their water than on their family income (Figure 2.5) [35]. The prevalence of *H. pylori* was 62% in low-income families using an external tap compared with 39% in those with a tap in the home. All the high-income families had a tap in their homes, but the prevalence of infection was 37% if they drank municipal water compared with only 4% if they drank water from a well. Worldwide, contaminated water may often be ingested when it is taken as a drink. Alternatively foods may become contaminated if they are irrigated with dirty

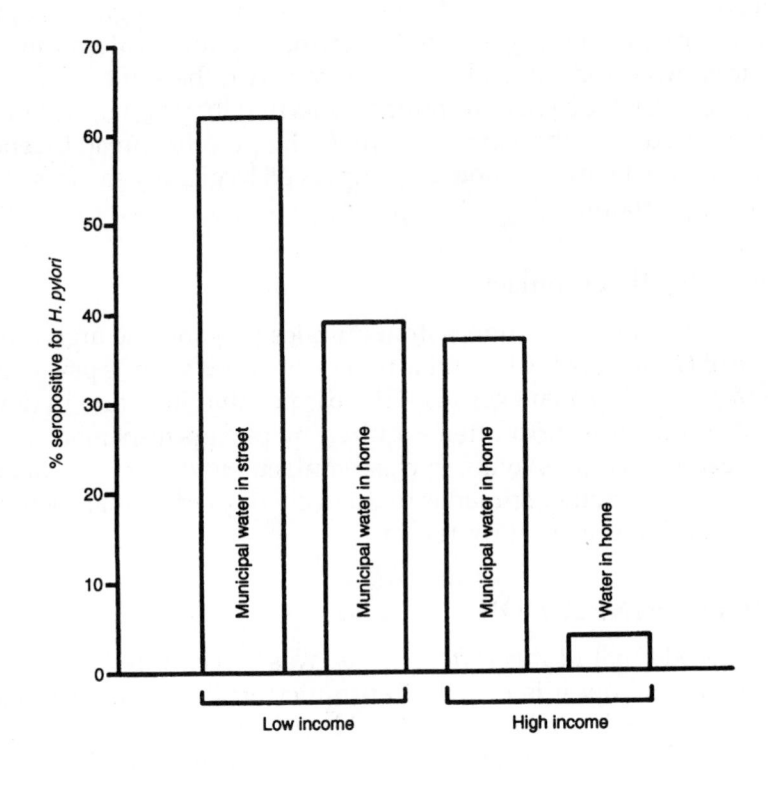

Figure 2.5 The prevalence of *H. pylori* in children in a village in Peru depended on the family income, but more on the source of water in the home. (*Source*: from data in reference 35.)

water, or if they are washed in it. This might explain why infection rates in part of Chile were higher in people who ate uncooked, rather than cooked vegetables [34].

In the West water does not appear to be an important mode of spread for infections in general or *H. pylori* in particular. A study in a small town and surrounding rural regions in Germany showed no correlation between the prevalence of *H. pylori* infection and the source of drinking water [36] .

Infection by gastric intubation

Infection has undoubtedly been spread by gastric intubation performed for research purposes, resulting in 'epidemics of achlorhydria' [37,38] (see below). There is also evidence that this infection has been spread between patients during diagnostic upper endoscopy [39]. Fingerprinting of strains in patients attending one clinic showed that several were infected with the same strain. The only thing that they had in common was that they had been serially endoscoped with the same instrument. Hopefully spread by endoscopy is now being prevented by improved hygiene measures in the endoscopy room.

Spread by direct contact

The clustering of infection within families [17] and the high prevalence of *H. pylori* in the inhabitants of institutions such as psychiatric units [40] and orphanages [41,42] indicates that infection in developed countries is most often acquired by person-to-person spread between individuals living in close contact. However it is not altogether clear whether spread is exclusively or predominantly by the faecal–oral or oral–oral route.

ROUTE OF INFECTION

It seems odd that 12 years after *H. pylori* was first cultured there is still debate as to how it is usually transmitted in the West. One major problem is that it is only acquired by 1 in 200–300 Western persons per year (see above), so it is difficult to observe transmission taking place.

Oral–oral or faecal–oral?

Opinion is divided as to whether the infecting dose usually leaves the infected person through their mouth or their anus. Until recently the oral–oral route was favoured. Lee argued that transmission occurs between dogs, which vomit and lick each other's faces, but not between rats, which eat each other's faeces [43]. Gastro-oesophageal reflux may bring the bacteria from the stomach to the mouth, and oral spread may be facilitated by *H. pylori* colonizing the periodontal spaces. Spread might be facilitated by practices such as mothers chewing their babies' food before feeding it to them. Also, Chinese persons in Melbourne who dipped their chopsticks into a communal rice bowl were more likely to be infected than those who used separate bowls [44]. Unfortunately this evidence is not conclusive because these practices could merely be markers for people with unclean habits which increase spread by some other route. The concept of oral–oral spread has been examined more seriously by trying to detect the bacteria by culture or by using the polymerase chain reaction (PCR) to detect its DNA in saliva or periodontal scrapings from persons with *H. pylori* in their stomachs. Studies using PCR suggest that about 50% of infected persons have *H. pylori* in their mouths, and most often in the periodontal spaces [45,46], but there are two problems. Firstly, PCR might detect the DNA of other bacteria. Thus Megraud now recommends that at least two specific regions of *H. pylori*'s genome should be successfully amplified before the diagnosis is regarded as proven (Chapter 4). Secondly, this method does not distinguish between live bacteria and DNA from dead ones. For example *H. pylori* was detected by PCR in the gastric juice of 12 out of 13 infected persons [45] whereas most groups can only culture *H. pylori* from a minority of samples of gastric juice. Culture of oral samples should provide the answer but unfortunately the percentage of patients with culturable *H. pylori* in their mouth has varied from 0–100% in different studies. Ferguson *et al.* only managed to culture *H. pylori* from the saliva of one out of nine persons with gastric *H. pylori* [47]. That person had the same strain in the mouth and stomach. Oral–oral spread of *H. pylori* probably does occur occasionally, but the evidence now favours faecal–oral spread.

The concept of faecal–oral spread became enormously more plausible when Thomas *et al.* succeeded in culturing *H. pylori* from human faeces in 1992. Remarkably, the bacterium was grown from the faeces of nine out of 23 children aged 3–27 months in a village in the Gambia [48]. This finding, together with the contrast between spread within families [17] with children *versus* no spread between childless couples [18] in the West (see above), suggests that infected children are an important vector. It is currently unclear why this is so. Infected children might excrete more bacteria in their stools than infected adults. Fox found *H. mustelae* in the stools of ferrets more often when their gastric acid secretion was suppressed than when acid secretion was normal [49]. Thus children might excrete more *H. pylori* during first infection when acid secretion is low. In addition children may spread the infection because they pay less attention to hygiene or because as infants they do not defecate straight into the toilet.

There is general agreement that the bacterium enters the stomach via the mouth. Self-infection studies provide a hint of the conditions conducive to colonization [50]. Two people infected themselves successfully by drinking 1 000 000 000 and 300 000 bacteria respectively with antacids. However infection did not occur in a third researcher who took 40 000 000 bacteria fasting, without antacids, when the intragastric pH was 1.7. Therefore infection may be more likely if the intragastric pH is high. This normally occurs after meals, because food buffers the gastric contents.

IMPLICATIONS OF EPIDEMIOLOGICAL FINDINGS IN CLINICAL PRACTICE

Overall the findings indicate a need to improve sanitation in developing countries and to eliminate poverty, war and overcrowding. While we wait for this Utopia it would be particularly useful to have a way of decreasing rates of infection in young children, because they seem to be important vectors. This is feasible by a programme of screening and treating children. On the other hand, it would be ideal to have an effective vaccine.

Practice in developed countries

The findings indicate the need for scrupulous hygiene during upper gastrointestinal investigations to prevent infection of the staff and patients. One clinical question is whether to eradicate *H. pylori* from the family of a duodenal ulcer patient, as well as the patient himself, in order to prevent re-infection. In this context the results indicate that re-infection from within the family is unlikely unless they are under-privileged, or the household contains young children.

Practice in developing countries

The high infection and re-infection rates in poor areas of the world have profound implications for clinical practice, which need to be worked out. If ulcer patients rapidly become re-infected it may be safer to maintain them on long-term acid suppressant therapy, or to give repeated courses of a *Helicobacter*-suppressing agent such as bismuth, rather than relying on eradication therapy.

REFERENCES

1. Feldman RA. Prevention of *Helicobacter pylori* infection. In: Calam J, ed. *Baillière's Clinical Gastroenterology: Helicobacter pylori.* London: Baillière Tindall, 1995: **9**: 447–465.
2. Graham DY, Malaty HM, Evans DG *et al.* Epidemiology of *Helicobacter pylori* in an asymptomatic population in the United States. Effect of age, race, and socioeconomic status. *Gastroenterology* 1991; **100**: 1495–1501.
3. Anonymous. Epidemiology of, and risk factors for, *Helicobacter pylori* infection among 3194 asymptomatic subjects in 17 populations. The EUROGAST Study Group. *Gut* 1993; **34**: 1672–1676.
4. Mathialagan R, Loizou S, Beales ILP *et al.* Who gets false-negative *H. pylori* (HP) ELISA results? (abstract). *Gut* 1994; **35**(suppl 5): S1.
5. Parsonnet J, Blaser MJ, Perez Perez GI *et al.* Symptoms and risk factors of *Helicobacter pylori* infection in a cohort of epidemiologists. *Gastroenterology* 1992; **102**: 41–46.
6. Kuipers EJ, Pena AS, Van Kamp G *et al.* Seroconversion for *Helicobacter pylori. Lancet* 1993; **342**: 328–331.
7. Banatvala N, Mayo K, Megraud F *et al.* The cohort effect and *Helicobacter pylori. J Infect Dis* 1993; **168**: 219–221.
8. Smoak BL, Kelley PW, Taylor DN. Seroprevalence of *Helicobacter pylori* infections in a cohort of US Army recruits. *Am J Epidemiol* 1994; **139**: 513–519.
9 Megraud F, Brassens Rabbe MP, Denis F *et al.* Seroepidemiology of *Campylobacter pylori* infection in various populations. *J Clin Microbiol* 1989; **27**: 1870–1873.
10. Anonymous. Ecology of *Helicobacter pylori* in Peru: infection rates in coastal, high altitude, and jungle communities. Gastrointestinal Physiology Working Group of the Cayetano Heredia and the Johns Hopkins University. *Gut* 1992; **33**: 604–605.
11. Correa P, Fox J, Fontham E *et al. Helicobacter pylori* and gastric carcinoma. Serum antibody prevalence in populations with contrasting cancer risks. *Cancer* 1990; **66**: 2569–2574.

12. Graham DY, Adam E, Reddy GT *et al.* Seroepidemiology of *Helicobacter pylori* infection in India. Comparison of developing and developed countries. *Dig Dis Sci* 1991; **36**: 1084–1088.

13. Coelho LG, Passos MC, Chausson Y *et al.* Duodenal ulcer and eradication of *Helicobacter pylori* in a developing country. An 18-month follow-up study. *Scand J Gastroenterol* 1992; **27**: 362–366.

14. Fiedorek SC, Malaty HM, Evans DL *et al.* Factors influencing the epidemiology of *Helicobacter pylori* infection in children. *Pediatrics* 1991; **88**: 578–582.

15. Webb PM, Knight T, Greaves S *et al.* Relation between infection with *Helicobacter pylori* and living conditions in childhood: evidence for person to person transmission in early life. *Br Med J* 1994; **308**: 750–753.

16. Mendall MA, Goggin PM, Molineaux N *et al.* Childhood living conditions and *Helicobacter pylori* seropositivity in adult life. *Lancet* 1992; **339**: 896–897.

17. Drumm B, Perez Perez GI, Blaser MJ, Sherman PM. Intrafamilial clustering of *Helicobacter pylori* infection. *N Engl J Med* 1990; **322**: 359–363.

18. Perez Perez GI, Witkin SS, Decker MD, Blaser MJ. Sero-prevalence of *Helicobacter pylori* infection in couples. *J Clin Microbiol* 1991; **29**: 642–644.

19. Nwokolo CU, Bickley J, Attard AR *et al.* Evidence of clonal variants of *Helicobacter pylori* in three generations of a duodenal ulcer disease family. *Gut* 1992; **33**: 1323–1327.

20. Mitchell HM, Lee A, Carrick J. Increased incidence of *Campylobacter pylori* infection in gastroenterologists: further evidence to support person-to-person transmission of *C. pylori*. *Scand J Gastroenterol* 1989; **24**: 396–400.

21. Hammermeister I, Janus G, Schamarowski F *et al.* Elevated risk of *Helicobacter pylori* infection in submarine crews. *Eur J Clin Microbiol Infect Dis* 1992; **11**: 9–14.

22. Thomas JE, Austin S, Dale A *et al.* Protection by human milk IgA against *Helicobacter pylori* infection in infancy (letter). *Lancet* 1993; **342**: 121.

23. Handt LK, Fox JG, Dewhirst FE *et al. Helicobacter pylori* isolated from the domestic cat: public health implications. *Infect Immun* 1994; **62**: 2367–2374.

24. Thomson MA, Storey P, Greer R, Cleghorn GJ. Canine–human transmission of *Gastrospirillum hominis*. *Lancet* 1994; **343**: 1605–1607.

25. Vaira D, D'Anastasio C, Holton J *et al. Campylobacter pylori* in abattoir workers: is it a zoonosis? *Lancet* 1988; **ii**: 725–726.
26. Vaira D, D'Anastasio C, Holton J *et al.* Is *Campylobacter pylori* a zoonosis? (letter). *Lancet* 1988; **ii**: 1149.
27. Goodwin S, Armstrong J, Bronsdon M, Sly L. Is *Campylobacter pylori* a zoonosis? (letter). *Lancet* 1988; **ii**: 968.
28. Correa P, Cuello C, Fajardo LF *et al.* Diet and gastric cancer: nutrition survey in a high-risk area. *J Natl Cancer Inst* 1983; **70**: 673–678.
29. Karim QN, Maxwell RH. Survival of *Campylobacter pylori* in artificially contaminated milk (letter). *J Clin Pathol* 1989; **42**: 778.
30. Hopkins RJ, Russell RG, O'Donnoghue JM *et al.* Seroprevalence of *Helicobacter pylori* in Seventh-Day Adventists and other groups in Maryland. Lack of association with diet. *Arch Intern Med* 1990; **150**: 2347–2348.
31. Webberley MJ, Webberley JM, Newell DG *et al.* Sero-epidemiology of *Helicobacter pylori* infection in vegans and meat-eaters. *Epidemiol Infect* 1992; **108**: 457–462.
32. Shahamat M, Mai U, Paszko Kolva C *et al.* Use of autoradio-graphy to assess viability of *Helicobacter pylori* in water. *Appl Environ Microbiol* 1993; **59**: 1231–1235.
33. West AP, Millar MR, Tompkins DS. Effect of physical environment on survival of *Helicobacter pylori. J Clin Pathol* 1992; **45**: 228–231.
34. Hopkins RJ, Vial PA, Ferreccio C *et al.* Seroprevalence of *Helicobacter pylori* in Chile: vegetables may serve as one route of transmission. *J Infect Dis* 1993; **168**: 222–226.
35. Klein PD, Graham DY, Gaillour A, Opekun AR, Smith EO. Water source as risk factor for *Helicobacter pylori* infection in Peruvian children. Gastrointestinal Physiology Working Group. *Lancet* 1991; **337**: 1503–1506.
36. Nowottny U, Heilmann KL. [Epidemiology of *Helicobacter pylori* infection]. *Leber Magen Darm* 1990; **20**: 180, 183–86.
37. Ramsey EJ, Carey KV, Peterson WL *et al.* Epidemic gastritis with hypochlorhydria. *Gastroenterology* 1979; **76**: 1449–1457.
38. Graham DY, Alpert LC, Smith JL, Yoshimura HH. Iatrogenic *Campylobacter pylori* infection is a cause of epidemic achlorhydria. *Am J Gastroenterol* 1988; **83**: 974–980.
39. Kosunen TU, Hook J, Rautelin HI, Myllyla G. Age-dependent increase of *Campylobacter pylori* antibodies in blood donors. *Scand J Gastroenterol* 1989; **24**: 110–114.

40. Berkowicz J, Lee A. Person-to-person transmission of *Campylobacter pylori* (letter). *Lancet* 1987; **ii**: 680–681.
41. Perez Perez GI, Taylor DN, Bodhidatta L *et al.* Seroprevalence of *Helicobacter pylori* infections in Thailand. *J Infect Dis* 1990; **161**: 1237–1241.
42. Reiff A, Jacobs E, Kist M. Seroepidemiological study of the immune response to *Campylobacter pylori* in potential risk groups. *Eur J Clin Microbiol Infect Dis* 1989; **8**: 592–596.
43. Lee A, Fox JG, Otto G *et al.* Transmission of *Helicobacter* spp. A challenge to the dogma of faecal–oral spread. *Epidemiol Infect* 1991; **107**: 99–109.
44. Chow THF, Lambert JR, Walquist ML, Hage BH. The influence of chopstick culture on the epidemiology of *Helicobacter pylori* – a study of two representative populations in Melbourne (abstract). *Gastroenterology* 1992; **120**: A605.
45. Mapstone NP, Lynch DA, Lewis FA *et al.* Identification of *Helicobacter pylori* DNA in the mouths and stomachs of patients with gastritis using PCR. *J Clin Pathol* 1993; **46**: 540–543.
46. Song M, Detection of *Helicobacter pylori* in human saliva by using nested polymerase chain reaction. *Chung Hua Liu Hsing Ping Hsueh Tsa Chih* 1993; **14**: 237–240.
47. Ferguson DA Jr, Li C, Patel NR *et al.* Isolation of *Helicobacter pylori* from saliva. *J Clin Microbiol* 1993; **31**: 2802–2804.
48. Thomas JE, Gibson GR, Darboe MK *et al.* Isolation of *Helicobacter pylori* from human faeces. *Lancet* 1992; **340**: 1194–1195.
49. Fox JG, Blanco MC, Yan L *et al.* Role of gastric pH in isolation of *Helicobacter mustelae* from the feces of ferrets. *Gastroenterology* 1993; **104**: 86–92.
50. Morris AJ, Ali MR, Nicholson GI *et al.* Long-term follow-up of voluntary ingestion of *Helicobacter pylori*. *Ann Intern Med* 1991; **114**: 662–663.

3

Disease associations

INTRODUCTION

This chapter will discuss the several diseases that *H. pylori* is proved, or suspected, to cause. Two aspects impress: firstly, that this discovery has changed our perception of these diseases totally; secondly, that *H. pylori* causes different diseases in different people. Therefore, for each disease, it is interesting to ask not only *whether H. pylori* causes it, but also *why* the disease occurs in that particular person. Dixon has studied the histopathology of *H. pylori* infection, and recently written an excellent review of it [1].

FIRST INFECTION

Introduction

This is a strange topic because much of what we know of it is based on observations made before the discovery of *H. pylori*. According to Marshall [2], these reports date from the 1920 edition of Osler's Textbook of Medicine. This describes gastritis with dyspepsia, flatulence, vomiting and hypochlorhydric gastric juice in the children of London [2]. In addition we have quite detailed data from a small number of researchers who infected themselves or their subjects, either through thirst for knowledge or lack of care.

Histology

Microscopy shows degeneration of the surface epithelium with mucin depletion, exfoliation of surface cells with compensatory foveolar hyperplasia. Neutrophils are present throughout the lamina propria of the antrum and corpus and infiltrating the surface and foveolar epithelia (Plate 1). Histologists use the terms 'acute' and 'active' when they see neutrophil polymorphs and 'chronic' when chronic inflammatory cells, predominantly lymphocytes and plasma cells, move in. In this sense *H. pylori* gastritis becomes chronic after only 1–2 weeks.

Pathogenesis

The earliest changes are likely to be due to bacterial products. Several candidates have been identified but it is difficult to dissect which is most important. Only about 60% of strains produce vacuolating toxin so other factors must be considered. Ammonia from *H. pylori*'s urease can cause mucosal damage by itself but is also an important ingredient for the production of monochloramine, which is more toxic [3]. Monochloramine is produced when ammonia reacts with chloride ions in the presence of oxygen free radicals formed by neutrophils. *H. pylori* also produces a phospholipase which can digest the protective mucus layer as well as cell membranes themselves [4]. Finally, *H. pylori* either makes platelet activating factor (PAF) itself or causes mast cells to release it [5]. Activation of platelets by PAF is likely to thrombose mucosal capillaries leading to local hypoxia. *H. pylori*'s endotoxin might also cause microthrombosis by causing endothelial damage. Neutrophil polymorphs may be attracted into the gastric mucosa by bacterial chemotaxins (Chapter 1) or by host responses such as complement activation and the expression of cytokines such as IL-8 [6]. Mucosal immunocytes produce IgA and IgM antibodies directed against *H. pylori* antigens in acute *H. pylori* gastritis [7].

Pathophysiology

A striking feature of first infection with *H. pylori* is that acid secretion more or less disappears for a few months, before gradually reappearing [8] (Figure 3.1). This was first observed by gastric physiologists who inadvertently cross-infected their subjects by not disinfecting their gastric tubes properly. Retrospective analysis of stored sera showed the appearance of antibodies to *H. pylori* at this time [9]. The loss of acid could be regarded teleologically as helping the infection to become established. Loss of acid secretion could be due to bacterial factors or to the host's response. Cave and Vargas reported that a product of *Helicobacter* inhibits uptake of aminopyrine, a marker of acid secretion, into parietal cells [10]. The factor responsible is currently being characterized. Another possibility is

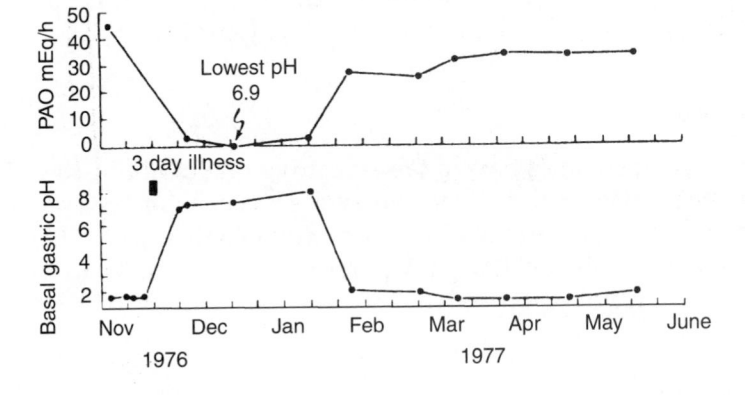

Figure 3.1 'Epidemic achlorhydria' due to first infection with *H. pylori*. PAO = peak acid output. Note that acid secretion returns after about 3 months. (*Source*: from reference 8, with permission.)

that epithelial degeneration leads to back-diffusion of any acid that is produced. On the other hand, *H. pylori* infection leads to release of a variety of cytokines, including interleukin-1-beta [11]. Infusions of this suppress acid secretion in rats [12] so it might be the cytokines released in acute *H. pylori* gastritis that cause the loss of acid secretion. In this respect it is of interest that acid secretion also disappears during severe infections such as typhoid, paratyphoid, pulmonary tuberculosis, bronchopneumonia and lung abscess [13].

Endoscopic appearances [14]

Macroscopic abnormalities are mainly seen in the antrum but may also involve the corpus. The spectrum of endoscopic appearances ranges from a purulent exudative gastritis to a pseudo-tumour appearance, erosions or ulcers, but in other patients there may be little to be seen. Resolution occurs within 2–4 weeks.

Symptoms [14]

First infection can be entirely symptom-free, but some patients develop a clinical syndrome known outside the medical profession as 'gastric flu'. There may be epigastric colic, nausea, vomiting, flatulence, malaise and in some cases fever. These symptoms persist for about 1–2 weeks. Acute gastric ulceration can present with haemorrhage. Loss of acid secretion led to a paradoxical improvement in a patient with the Zollinger–Ellison syndrome [15].

Outcome

Most serological tests have a false-positive rate of about 10%. This might be partly due to patients who were recently infected but have spontaneously cleared their infection. However it appears that once infection is established it usually persists for decades or even for life if treatment is not given.

Management

Infection may be diagnosed and treated in the usual way, but bearing in mind that the serological response during the first week or so is likely to be with IgM and IgA rather than IgG. Diminished acid secretion is likely to increase the chance of successful eradication. This may be one reason why eradication rates tend to be higher in children than in adults (Chapter 6). However, Morris, having deliberately infected himself, failed to eradicate the bacteria on his first attempt [7].

CHRONIC GASTRITIS

Most people with *H. pylori* infection have an asymptomatic chronic gastritis without ulcers, cancer or lymphoma. This condition is nevertheless important because individuals with it are quite strongly predisposed to these more serious conditions.

Histology

The classification of chronic gastritis: a short history
It is necessary to understand how the classification of gastritis has evolved in order to make sense of the literature. Before the discovery of *H. pylori*, chronic non-specific gastritis was a frustrating topic to study. Its association with more serious gastroduodenal diseases was well recognized but its role in these conditions and its aetiology were uncertain. These aspects made chronic gastritis difficult to classify. Faber first pointed out the difference between the superficial

and atrophic forms of chronic gastritis in 1927 [16]. Chronic superficial gastritis implies an increase in chronic inflammatory cells in the
superficial part of the lamina propria. Chronic atrophic gastritis has
come to mean that there is glandular atrophy **and** chronic inflammatory cells throughout the mucosa. Confusion arises because some
patients have glandular atrophy with scanty or absent chronic cells,
as in pernicious anaemia, or full-thickness chronic cells without
glandular atrophy, the so-called 'interstitial' or 'pre-atrophic'
gastritis.

Classifications based on the regions of the stomach affected (topography) and clinical associations initially brought some clarity, but
then became over-complicated. In 1973 Strickland and Mackay
pointed out two major categories of chronic gastritis with atrophy
[17]. Type A is the pattern seen in patients with pernicious anaemia.
These patients have parietal cell autoantibodies, predominant in-
volvement of the corpus and drastically decreased acid secretion.
Type B gastritis lacked parietal cell autoantibodies and mainly
affected the antrum. The aetiology of this type remained obscure
and bile reflux, therapeutic drugs, hot drinks and salty or spicy food
were all suggested. In 1975 Glass and Pitchumoni added type AB
chronic gastritis. Patients with this had patchy gastritis and atrophy
in both the corpus and antrum [18]. This pattern of gastritis is now
called multifocal atrophy. It is associated with intestinal metaplasia
and carries an increased risk of gastric ulcers and cancer.

It is now appreciated that *H. pylori* is responsible for the diffuse
antral gastritis associated with duodenal and prepyloric ulcers.
Indeed, this bacterium probably causes the great majority of non-
autoimmune gastritis worldwide. However, communication and
comparison of results was still hampered by differences in classification, partly resulting from the different patterns of gastritis seen
in different countries of the world.

The Sydney system was devised to remove ambiguities by pro-
viding a simple statement of what is seen in the gastric antrum and
corpus [19]. Neutrophils, chronic cells, glandular atrophy, intestinal
metaplasia and *H. pylori* are all graded on a four-point scale of
normal, mild, moderate or severe. Special forms of gastritis are
considered separately and not subject to grading.

Histological features of chronic H. pylori gastritis (Plate 2)
Epithelial degeneration and adhesion of bacteria
Epithelial degeneration is milder and more variable in the chronic
than in the acute phase of *H. pylori* gastritis. The amount of

degeneration in individual patients correlates with the percentage of bacteria that is adherent to the gastric epithelium [20]. Adhesion probably facilitates degeneration by enabling bacterial products to enter epithelial cells. Adhesion involves the bacterial adhesins, which vary from strain to strain, binding to epithelial receptors, which vary from person to person. Interestingly the epithelial receptors include the Lewis (b) blood group antigen, particularly if it is associated with blood group O [21]. About 80% of the population secrete blood group substances in their saliva and gastric juice. This might decrease adhesion by saturating the bacterium's receptors in the gastric lumen. The amount of epithelial degeneration also correlates with the density of infiltration by neutrophil polymorphs.

Neutrophil polymorphs
The terms 'active' and 'acute' are used to indicate that neutrophil polymorphs are present. These infiltrate the lamina propria and also the epithelium itself. Their presence correlates with epithelial degeneration, which is not surprising because neutrophils release several injurious products. Neutrophils may be attracted by bacterial chemotaxis as well as cytokines such as IL8 released in the inflamed mucosa. Neutrophils generally persist throughout life but their numbers may diminish in older people with marked glandular atrophy. This tends to occur over the age of 70 years in the West, but earlier in countries where childhood infection is the rule [22].

Chronic inflammatory cells
Gastritis is regarded as chronic when chronic inflammatory cells – lymphocytes and plasma cells – are present. Normal uninfected mucosa contains scattered aggregates of lymphocytes, deep in the mucosa of the gastric corpus, close to the muscularis mucosae, but these are not normally present in the antrum. Chronic gastritis is diagnosed when any lymphocytes, however few, are present in the superficial part of the lamina propria. The degree of chronic inflammatory infiltrate correlates closely with the extent and density of *H. pylori* colonization and is thus generally more severe in the antrum [23].

Mechanisms

Detailed immunology is beyond the scope of this book and there have been several excellent reviews [24–27]. Certain aspects are described here because they give a clue to the sort of factors that might lead to different disease outcomes. Chronic inflammation is probably a response to *H. pylori* antigens so bacterial heterogeneity is one factor that may contribute to differences between patients. Bacterial antigens include the enzyme urease [28], endotoxin [29] (i.e. lipopolysaccharide), 62 kDa heat shock protein [30], 87 kDa vacuolating toxin [31] and 120–128 kDa CagA product [32] (Chapter 1). Non-toxigenic strains typically lack the last two of these and produce milder inflammation. When gastrointestinal epithelia become inflamed the epithelial cells take on some of the characteristics normally associated with monocytes. For example, they release cytokines in the same way that monocytes do [33]. Cytokines are many and varied but their overall effect is to attract and activate leucocytes. Heterogeneity of the immune response is particularly likely to affect disease outcomes. Class II molecules, including HLA antigens, are expressed on epithelial cells [34] in *H. pylori* gastritis as well as monocytes. Their function is to present antigens to the immune system, so it is not surprising that variation in HLA type produces different disease outcomes. Both we [35] and a Japanese group [36] have found associations between specific HLA-DQ types and disease outcomes in *H. pylori* infection. Once presented with antigens the B-lymphocytes produce IgM, secretory IgA, and IgG antibodies against *H. pylori*. Secretory IgA may play a blocking role, reducing bacterial adhesion and complement activation, but IgG is probably most important in the mucosal immune response. IgG antibodies promote complement-dependent phagocytosis and killing of bacteria by polymorphs. Other inflammatory mediators released by monocytes and polymorphs include prostaglandins, leucotrienes, proteases and reactive oxygen species [37]. The last may be a particularly important cause of tissue damage but are inactivated by *H. pylori*'s catalase and by the antioxidant vitamins C and E. It has recently been shown that vitamin C is actively secreted into the gastric lumen, but that this secretion is decreased in *H. pylori* infection [38]. Tissue concentrations of alpha-tocopherol (vitamin E) are also decreased in actively inflamed corpus mucosa [39]. Thus it is easy to see how the amount of oxidative damage could depend on aspects of the bacterial strain and the host that determine the number and activity of neutrophils on the one hand and the patient's nutritional status on the other. In this context it is interesting that a low intake of antioxidant vitamins increases the risk of gastric cancer [40]. Neutrophil polymorphs tend to gather around the proliferative compartment of the pit isthmus where stem cells are located.

Damage to these cells by neutrophil products may therefore contribute to the cellular changes seen in glandular atrophy.

Lymphoid follicles (Plate 3)

The lymphocytes attracted into the gastric mucosa by *H. pylori* were always interesting with respect to immunological responses, but have recently gained far greater importance with the discovery that this infection predisposes to gastric lymphomas [41]. Uninfected gastric mucosa contains scanty lymphocytes close to the muscularis mucosae in the corpus, but infected mucosa usually [42] or perhaps always [43] contains aggregates of B-cells with germinal centres. Lymphoid follicles are prominent in children infected with *H. pylori*, leading to their characteristic nodular antral gastritis [44]. These lymphoid follicles are an example of acquired mucosa-associated lymphoid tissue (MALT). As *H. pylori* results in acquisition of MALT, it is likely to be a key factor in the development of gastric B-cell lymphomas (MALTomas). In some cases the lymphoid nodules do expand and take on features of gastric lymphoma, with expansion of the lymphocyte population, larger follicles and lymphocytes invading epithelial structures [43]. After making a diagnosis of gastric lymphoma it is wise to try anti-helicobacter therapy, because some cases that satisfy the accepted criteria of malignant lymphoma have been successfully treated by eradication of *H. pylori* [45].

Atrophy (Plate 4)

Atrophy is a loss of glandular tissue which results from repeated tissue injury and leads to thinning of the gastric mucosa. The injury might be a focal lesion such as an ulcer, but chronic gastritis is a diffuse process which probably leads to piecemeal injury to glands. An important feature of atrophy is that restitution and regeneration, which should restore a normal mucosa, ceases to do so. One idea is that destruction of the basement membrane and the cells which support it prevents normal restitution. There is also an important change in the behaviour of gastric stem cells. Regeneration tends to produce metaplastic 'pseudo-pyloric' glands, containing cells of the 'ulcer-associated lineage' (UACL) (Plate 5) [46]. This probably aids repair by manufacturing growth factors. Those produced include epidermal growth factor (EGF) which inhibits acid secretion as well as stimulating epithelial growth.

In patients with chronic *H. pylori* gastritis the prevalence and severity of glandular atrophy increases steadily with age. Patients without *H. pylori* infection, or other forms of gastritis, rarely develop atrophy and secrete normal amounts of gastric acid into old age [47]. For example, Kuipers *et al.* found that 16 out of 56 infected persons developed atrophy over 12 years, compared with only two of 49 uninfected individuals [48]. *H. pylori* may be eliminated as atrophy progresses. This is because the gastric environment becomes less hospitable. The bacterium cannot adhere to gastric mucosa which has undergone intestinal metaplasia, and needs some acid to neutralize the alkali that it generates [49]. Therefore there is a group of older patients who have *H.-pylori*-related atrophy but are no longer infected [50].

H. pylori infection produces gastric atrophy in some individuals, but not in others. The factors which lead to this divergence are important because they probably affect the risk of gastric cancer. *H. pylori* infection causes the host to produce autoantibodies which may contribute to the process of atrophy [51]. Autoimmunity occurs because bacterial antigens such as heat-shock protein resemble antigens in the host's epithelium [52]. Factors which alter the host's immune response are therefore likely to be important. We found that infected patients with atrophy had HLA-DQ5 over three times more often than infected patients without atrophy or uninfected controls [35]. Certain HLA-DQ types are associated with diminished immune responses. We also found that infected patients with atrophy have less circulating IgG antibodies against *H. pylori* than infected patients without atrophy [53]. This might be because the bacterial load or the mucosal response is diminished in gastric atrophy. But it is also possible that a feeble immune response is conducive to atrophy. Patients with agammaglobulinaemia virtually always have severe atrophy and have 40 times the normal risk of gastric cancer [54].

Intestinal metaplasia (Plate 4)

Chronic gastritis frequently leads to intestinal metaplasia (IM). Its prevalence appears to reflect the duration and severity of inflammation. Worldwide, *H. pylori* is the commonest cause of chronic gastritis, but there are quite wide variations in the prevalence of IM between countries and ethnic groups. These differences presumably reflect differences in factors such as the age of acquisition, diet, and general health. *H. pylori* infection is more prevalent in individuals with IM than without it, despite the tendency of IM to clear the infection [55], suggesting that *H. pylori* is a major cause of IM. However bile reflux may also be important and research suggests that this acts synergistically with *H. pylori* to produce IM [56]. This is plausible because gastric mucosa which has been weakened by *H. pylori* is probably less able to withstand injury from refluxed bile. IM may start as a local temporary regenerative process, but chronic irritation leads to a more generalized and permanent change. Intestinal epithelium is resistant to bile and cannot be colonized by *H. pylori*, so the change is regarded by some as a protective adaptation. IM also tends to decrease the number of chronic inflammatory cells in the gastric mucosa [57]. Why gastric stem cells start to differentiate differently is not well understood. However the question is important because the development of IM is presumably an important step in the development of the intestinal type of cancer (see below).

Topography (Figure 3.2)

The distribution of gastritis within the stomach is interesting because different patterns of gastritis are seen in patients with different *H. pylori*-related diseases. Most cases of chronic *H. pylori* gastritis affect the whole stomach, but some patients have an antrum-predominant gastritis and these are more likely to develop duodenal or prepyloric ulcers. It seems likely that the relative lack of corpus gastritis in duodenal ulcer (DU) patients contributes to their increased acid secretion. Conversely the robust acid secretion may make the corpus inhospitable to *H. pylori*. Thus the development of a DU may depend on how vigorously the corpus mucosa repels the infection. Patients in whom malnutrition and intercurrent infections prevent this may never recover completely from their initial hypochlorhydric pangastritis. Persistent infection of the corpus in these individuals might lead to further atrophy and eventually in some patients to a gastric ulcer or cancer [17,18,58].

Gastric metaplasia of the duodenum and DU disease (Plate 6)

Gastric metaplasia is the appearance of gastric-mucus-type cells in the **surface** of the duodenal mucosa. This is not to be confused with gastric heterotopia, which is full-thickness corpus-type mucosa appearing as small sessile nodules at endoscopy. Gastric metaplasia is uncommon in Western children but develops progressively so that

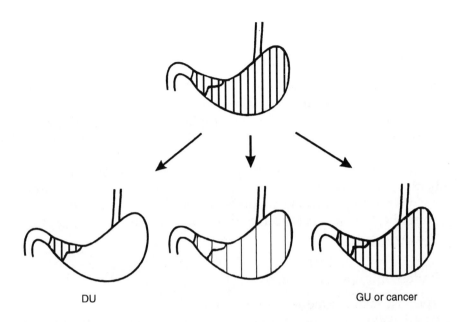

Figure 3.2 The topography of *H. pylori*-associated gastritis. First infection causes a severe pangastritis. Patients in whom chronic gastritis is more or less restricted to the gastric antrum are most likely to develop duodenal ulcer (DU) disease, while marked chronic pangastritis predisposes to gastric ulcer (GU) and gastric cancer. Patients with neither ulcers nor cancer can have either of these patterns but most often have a mild pangastritis. It is not known why different individuals develop these different patterns of gastritis.

it is present in a third of all adults undergoing endoscopy [59]. Gastric metaplasia is probably a non-specific response to injury because is also seen in patients with duodenal Crohn's disease. However it is most often a response to the duodenal acid load. It can be induced in animals by repeated injections of gastrin [60]. It is extensive in patients with gastrin-secreting tumours [61], but lacking in patients with achlorhydria [62]. The prevalence of gastric metaplasia is increased in patients with duodenal ulcer disease [63] but decreased after acid-lowering operations for this condition [64], suggesting that the process is slowly reversible. Gastric metaplasia correlates closely with the presence of duodenitis. It probably plays a vital role in the development of duodenal ulcers by allowing

H. pylori to colonize the duodenum and thus cause local injury to the mucosa.

Histological changes after eradication of *H. pylori*

Neutrophil polymorphs move out rapidly after eradication therapy and their disappearance is a useful histological marker of success. Surface degeneration also resolves rapidly. The number of chronic cells declines much more slowly so that it may take 6–12 months for mean scores to fall by 50%. Indeed the numbers of lymphocytes and plasma cells may never reach pre-infection levels. This might be because *H. pylori* initiates an ongoing autoimmune process. At present it is not altogether clear whether glandular atrophy is reversible on eradication of *H. pylori* but some preliminary reports suggest that it is [65].

Endoscopic appearances

The gastric mucosa often appears normal in chronic *H. pylori* gastritis. In other cases there are patches of erythema contrasting with whiter areas in between. The mucosa may be slightly uneven, with a loss of shininess. Occasionally there are tiny whitish spots of exudate together with small erosions, particularly in the prepyloric region. Rarely there is a more marked erosive gastritis of the distal stomach. A more characteristic appearance is the combination of antritis with inflammation of the duodenal bulb. *H. pylori* duodenitis produces punctate erythema and punctate or confluent erosions combined with mild oedema accentuating the pattern of mucosal folds [66].

Management

At present uncomplicated *H. pylori* gastritis is not generally regarded as an indication for eradication therapy. However once it is diagnosed the patients may request therapy and this is not unreasonable in view of the association with diseases, including gastric cancer. In this respect it would be interesting to know the effect of eradicating *H. pylori* at different ages on the subsequent risk of developing gastric cancer. This information will be difficult to obtain but reports that atrophy reverses following eradication are encouraging [65]. Another clinically important question is whether eradication of *H. pylori* improves dyspeptic symptoms in patients without ulcers (see below).

DUODENAL ULCER DISEASE

Introduction

The greatest clinical impact of the discovery of *H. pylori* has been in duodenal ulcer (DU) disease. Here medical research has made a common chronic clinical condition curable by a short course of treatment. We must thank Richard Warren and Barry Marshall for this remarkable achievement. The main task now it to ensure that as many DU patients as possible benefit from this breakthrough.

Definition and epidemiology

A duodenal ulcer (DU) is defined as a breach in the duodenal epithelium associated with acute and chronic inflammation. DUs are exceedingly common. A survey in Finland showed that 1.4% of the entire population have a DU at any time [67]. The lifetime prevalence of DU was 10% in males and 4% in females [68]. The number of new cases per year (the incidence) was about 0.2% in males and 0.1% in females [69]. In the United Kingdom DUs are more common in the north of the country and in urban rather than rural regions [68]. The incidence of DUs gradually rises with age but peaks at about 60 years of age. Much of the early and international data on the prevalence of duodenal ulcers are available only as observations of the ratio of DUs to gastric ulcers (GUs). The findings are nevertheless interesting. In most parts of the world DUs are about three times as common as GUs, but GUs are more common in some places such as Japan, Sri Lanka, the Andes and some islands off northern Norway.

A highly interesting aspect of ulcer epidemiology is that it is changing quite rapidly. William Brinton recorded in late 19th-century England that GUs occurred in young women and were much more common than DUs [70]. From the turn of the century until about 1960 the incidence of DU rose several times to become more common than GU, which is now uncommon under the age of 40 years. Since 1960 the incidence of DU has stopped rising and may even have declined [68]. In 1962 Susser and Stein suggested that the depression of the 1930s had created a cohort of individuals at risk of DU [71]. It is tempting to suggest that *H. pylori* was responsible for this increase in DUs. The change in the GUs is more difficult to explain, but presumably reflects altered environmental factors such as diet or drug ingestion, or perhaps a different strain of *H. pylori* has emerged.

Risk factors (Table 3.1)
The risk of DU disease is increased greatly by cigarette smoking [72] and slightly by therapy with non-steroidal anti-inflammatory drugs (NSAIDs) [73]. A moderate intake of alcohol is not harmful and may even decrease the risk of a DU [74], but DUs are considerably more common in patients with cirrhosis or pancreatitis, perhaps because they secrete less bicarbonate into the duodenum. Diet does not appear to have a marked effect in the West except that male college students who did not drink milk developed DUs more frequently than those who did [75]. A survey in India showed that DUs are much more prevalent in communities that eat rice than in communities that eat unrefined wheat. Furthermore the 5-year recurrence rate of DU was reduced from 84% to 14% when rice eaters were persuaded to eat wheat-based chapattis [76]. These data are generally

Table 3.1 Factors leading to specific disease outcomes in *H. pylori* infection

Duodenal ulcer	Gastric cancer
Generally accepted	• extensive gastric atrophy/ decreased parietal cell mass [183]
• cigarette smoking [72]	• diet:
• high parietal cell mass [89]/lack of corpus atrophy [103]	– low in antioxidant vitamins [40,183]
• duodenal metaplasia [63]	– high in salt [187]
• toxigenic strain of *H. pylori* [111,112]	• acquisition of *H. pylori* at less than 5 years of age [174]
• inherited factors [87]	• blood group A [191,193]
• male [68]	• toxigenic strain of *H. pylori* [194]
• blood group O and non-secretor [191]	• cigarette smoking [195]
	• humoral immunodeficiency [54]
Speculative	
• diet:	
– cola/coffee rather than milk [75]	
– rice rather than wheat [76]	
– no alcohol [74]	
• greater immune response to *H. pylori* [112]	
• acquisition of *H. pylori* at an older age	
• strains which activate neutrophils more strongly [192]	
• NSAIDs [73]	

interpreted in terms of the higher fibre content of wheat. However it is interesting that wheat leads to a loss of gastric acid secretion in patients with coeliac disease [77].

The evidence that H. pylori causes duodenal ulcers
It is now quite clear that *H. pylori* is the major cause of duodenal ulcers. The first evidence for this came from the observation that the human stomach often contains spiral bacteria (Chapter 1). This contradicted the general view that the stomach is normally sterilized by gastric acid. The next clue was the finding that healing DUs with the antibacterial agent bismuth produces longer remissions of DU disease than treatment with a histamine H_2-receptor antagonist [78]. However the picture only became clear with the observations of Warren and Marshall, which have proved to be entirely reproducible: firstly, that > 90% of DU patients were infected, compared with only about 40% of controls [79]; secondly, that eradication of *H. pylori* drastically reduces recurrence of DUs [80] (Figure 3.3). Indeed in most of the more recent studies, starting with the one in Amsterdam [81], the recurrence rate has been zero so the disease can be declared to be cured. Tytgat and Dixon have reviewed the effect of eradicating *H. pylori* on recurrence of DU in the various studies [82]. A few patients in the 'eradicated' group of early studies had recurrent DU. In retrospect, most of these patients probably had persisting infection. This is easily missed if eradication is not judged by a urease breath test done at least 1 month after the end of therapy. Recurrent duodenal ulceration does occur after successful eradication therapy at a rate which depends on how carefully patients with other conditions were excluded. Recurrent ulcers after successful eradication therapy may have another specific cause such as Crohn's disease, NSAID therapy or a gastrin-secreting tumour [83].

Effect of eradication on complications
Eradication of *H. pylori* drastically decreases the incidence of bleeding from peptic ulcers. Two studies examined the effect of eradication of *H. pylori* from patients with bleeding DUs and GUs. Rebleeding was 0% in those in whom the bacterium was eradicated compared with 38% and 28% respectively in those not successfully cleared of *H. pylori* [84,85]. Interestingly the prevalence of *H. pylori* in patients with perforated DUs appears to be no greater than in the general population [86]. If this is confirmed it suggests that perforation of the duodenum is actually due to a different disease process, such as ingestion of NSAIDs.

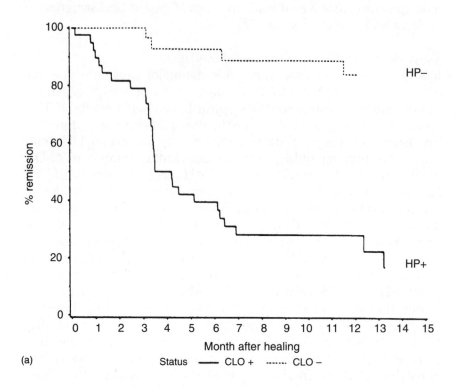

Figure 3.3 Two studies (above and opposite) showing the effect of eradicating *H. pylori* on recurrence of duodenal ulcers. Both show the percentage of patients remaining in remission after therapy which has (Hp–) or has not (Hp+) eradicated *H. pylori*. **(a)** shows the classical result obtained by Marshall *et al.* [80].

Disease mechanisms

Ideas before the discovery of H. pylori
Genetic or familial?
It is difficult to unravel genetic components from the familial spread of *H. pylori* in family studies. However there appears to be a genetic component, because concordance is higher in monozygotic than in dizygotic twins [87]. Candidate genes include those encoding HLA DQ which determines antigen presentation and blood groups related to bacterial adhesion.

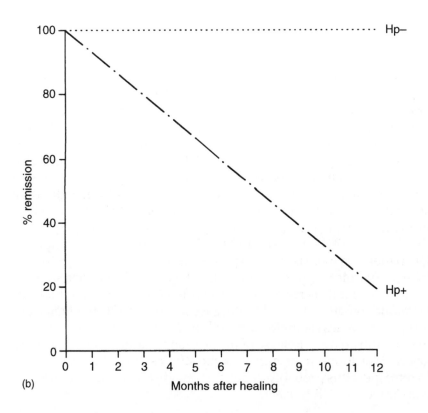

Figure 3.3 *continued* **(b)** shows the 'cure' of duodenal ulcer disease first reported by Rauws and Tytgat [81]. The latter presumably obtained 100% cure by diagnosing eradication accurately and by eliminating patients with ulcers due to other factors. (*Source*: redrawn from references 80 and 81, with permission.)

Psychological aspects
Folklore implicates stress in the aetiology of DU, but there is almost no evidence for this. The only evidence that I can find for this is that the incidence of perforated DUs increased during the Blitz of London [88]. This is plausible because psychological factors have many effects on gastrointestinal secretion, motility, blood flow and immunology. However, there are other possible explanations. The transmission of *H. pylori* might have been increased by wartime conditions (Chapter 2), although according to McColl's group, perforated ulcers are not due to *H. pylori* infection [86]. Also, the study was not controlled for cigarette smoking or the ingestion of analgesics.

Acid

The idea that *H. pylori* is the main cause of DUs was initially thought to contradict the previous hypothesis that acid secretion was important. However we now realize that *H. pylori* and acid interact in several ways in the pathogenesis of DUs. *H. pylori* only causes DUs in persons with a relatively high parietal cell mass. Secondly *H. pylori* affects gastric physiology in a way which increases acid secretion, and this might be an important ulcerogenic mechanism. Work before the discovery of *H. pylori* showed two main abnormalities of acid secretion in DU disease. Firstly DU patients have about twice the normal number of parietal cells [89] which gives them an elevated maximal acid output [90] (MAO) (Figure 3.4). Secondly they show defective reflex inhibition of acid secretion by factors such as intragastric acid [91,92] (Figure 3.5), gastric distension [93], intraduodenal fat [94] and fasting [89]. Meal-stimulated acid output in DU patients is increased in line with the MAO [89] but persists for longer after meals [92,95] (Figure 3.6). Physiological reflexes which normally inhibit secretion of acid involve release of the inhibitory hormone somatostatin within the gastric mucosa. DU patients were found to have less somatostatin cells and less somatostatin peptide in their antrum [96]. Release of the acid-stimulating antral hormone gastrin was found to be high in some studies but not in others [92]. In retrospect this probably depended on whether or not the controls were infected with *H. pylori*.

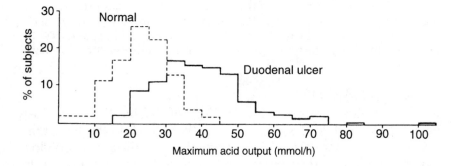

Figure 3.4 Graph showing the distribution of maximally stimulated acid output in patients with duodenal ulcers compared with normal controls. Maximal acid output is typically about 40 mmol/h in patients compared with about 20 mmol/h in controls, but there is considerable variation and overlap. (*Source*: from reference 90, with permission.)

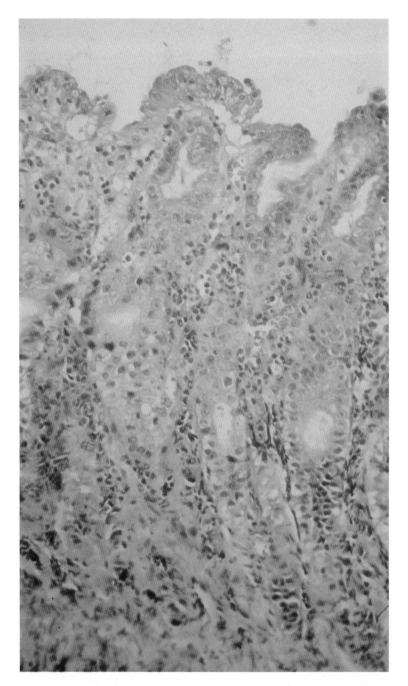

Plate 1 Gastric histology during first infection with *H. pylori*. Note the marked epithelial degeneration and the infiltrate of neutrophil polymorphs. (*Source*: provided by Dr M.F. Dixon.)

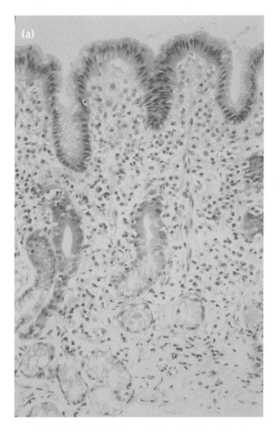

Plate 2 Two common patterns of *H. pylori*-associated chronic antral gastritis. In both cases the lamina propria is infiltrated with moderate numbers of chronic inflammatory cells. In (**b**) there is considerable epithelial surface damage and neutrophil infiltration but in (**a**) the surface is intact. The reason for this difference in damage is unclear but difference between the virulence of bacterial strains might be responsible. (*Source*: provided by Dr A.B. Price.)

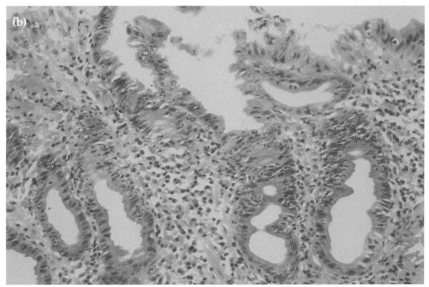

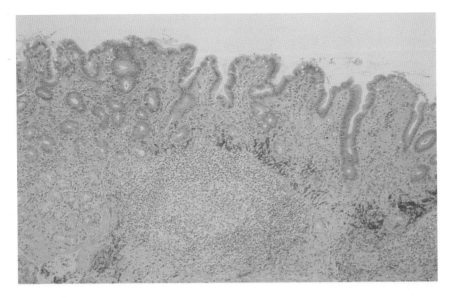

Plate 3 *H. pylori*-associated chronic antral gastritis showing prominent lymphoid hyperplasia in the lower half of the mucosa. Two follicles with large germinal centres are seen centre and left. (*Source*: provided by Dr A.B. Price.)

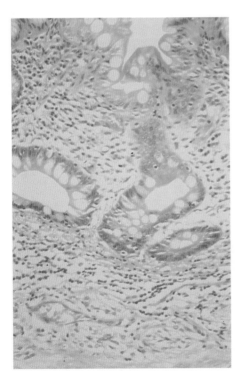

Plate 4 The full thickness of a gastric antral mucosal biopsy showing the loss of normal glands and replacement by intestinal metaplasia. There are large numbers of goblet cells, which appear vacuolated. This is chronic antral gastritis with severe atrophy and metaplasia. Atrophy and metaplasia usually occur together. (*Source*: provided by Dr A.B. Price.)

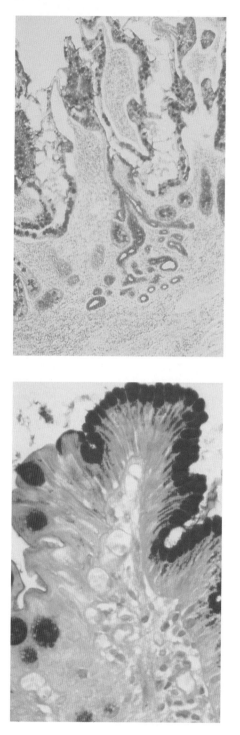

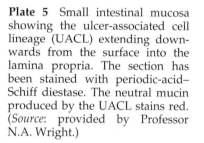

Plate 5 Small intestinal mucosa showing the ulcer-associated cell lineage (UACL) extending downwards from the surface into the lamina propria. The section has been stained with periodic-acid–Schiff diestase. The neutral mucin produced by the UACL stains red. (*Source*: provided by Professor N.A. Wright.)

Plate 6 In this duodenal biopsy the magenta-coloured gastric metaplasia contrasts with the blue goblet cells and brush border of the normal-coloured surface epithelium. (Periodic-acid–Schiff reagent and Alcian blue stain.) (*Source*: provided by Dr A.B. Price.)

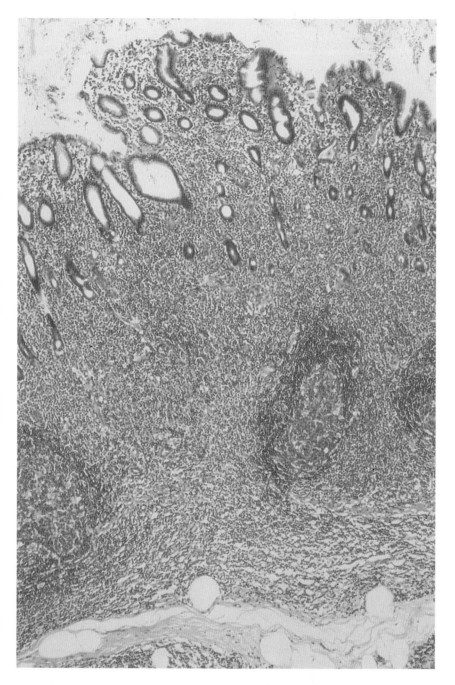

Plate 7 Gastric MALT lymphoma. Centrocyte-like cells with pale cytoplasm can be seen surrounding reactive lymphoid follicles and lympho-epithelial lesions can seen even at low power. (*Source*: provided by Dr A. Wotherspoon.)

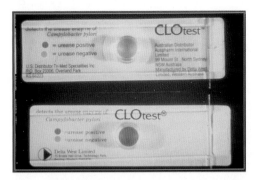

Plate 8 The CLO test®. The gel changes from orange to red after an infected biopsy is pushed into it.

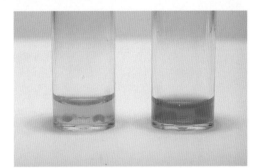

Plate 9 The biopsy urease test performed at low cost using McNulty's recipe.

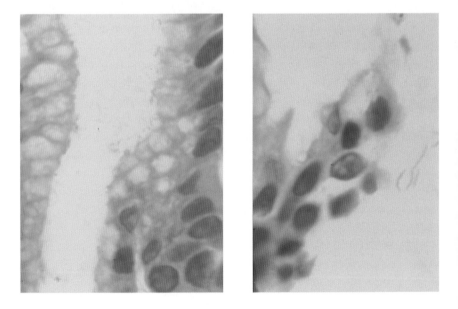

Plate 10 The contrast between the size and spiral configuration of *H. pylori* on the left and *H. heilmanii* (*Gastrospirillum hominis*) on the right. (H & E with oil immersion × 100.) (*Source*: provided by Dr A.B. Price.)

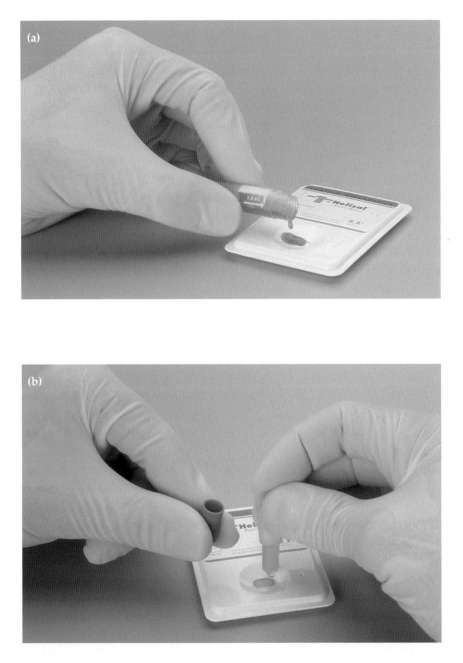

Plate 11 Diagnosis of *H. pylori* infection by Helisal™ Rapid Blood. (**a**) Finger-prick blood is mixed with buffer and poured into the well. (**b**) After this has filtered through the membrane the blue residue is wiped off and the second antibody is added. (**c**) and (**d**) *overleaf* The result is read after the second antibody has passed through. One dot indicates a negative result; two dots indicate a positive result.

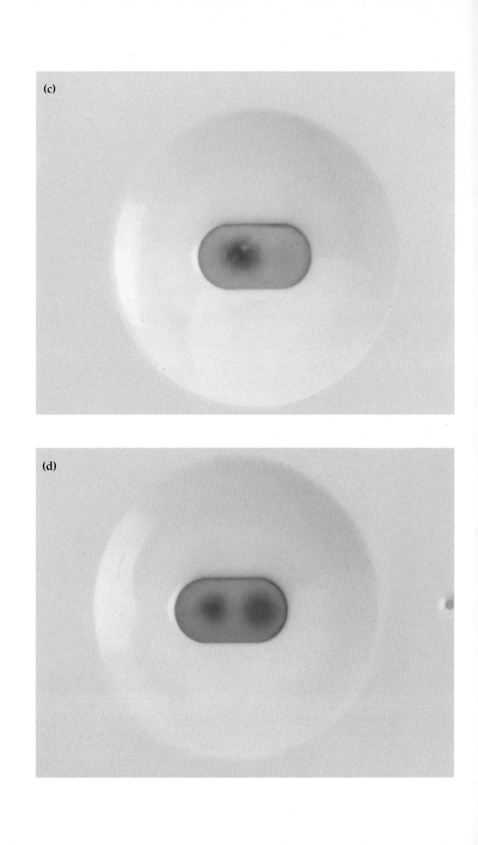

Gastrin and somatostatin: the effect of H. pylori

It is now clear that *H. pylori* is responsible for the abnormalities in the regulatory control of gastric function that were previously found when DU patients were compared with controls. Research by my

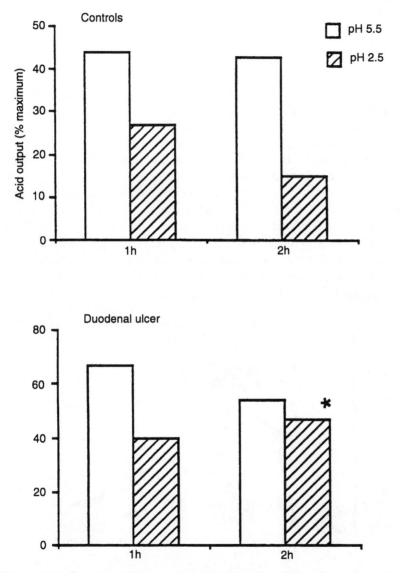

Figure 3.5 Gastric acid secretion stimulated by distending the stomach with a solution of peptone at a constant pH. Acid secretion is inhibited less by a low intragastric pH in patients with duodenal ulcers, suggesting a defect in inhibitory control. (*Source*: drawn from data in reference 91.)

group and others has shown that *H. pylori* increases plasma gastrin concentrations under all of the conditions which have been examined to date [92,97–99] (Figure 3.7) and decreases gastric mucosal expression of somatostatin mRNA [100] (Figure 3.8) and peptide [101].

Helicobacter pylori and gastric acid secretion

Under different conditions *H. pylori* can either increase or decrease gastric acid secretion: first infection leads to temporary achlorhydria [8,9] (see Figure 3.1). Chronic infection in subjects who do not have DUs causes atrophy of the gastric corpus mucosa, which leads to low acid output [102–104]. Effects of *H. pylori* on gastric physiology are revealed by controlling for these factors, either by studying DU patients who lack corpus atrophy [103] or by using patients as their own controls. Such studies show that *H. pylori* is responsible for the defective reflex inhibition of acid secretion that was previously noted in DU patients. Thus *H. pylori* increases acid secretion when the intragastric pH is low – during fasting [105] and during stimulation with meals [106] (Figure 3.9) or gastrin-releasing peptide [107] (Figure 3.10). This pattern of changes is explained by lack of the inhibitory peptide somatostatin (Figure 3.8). At present it is not clear whether the increased parietal cell mass in DU disease

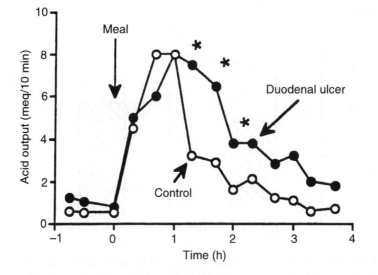

Figure 3.6 Meal-stimulated acid secretion is prolonged in patients with duodenal ulcers. (*Source*: redrawn from reference 95, with permission.)

is an inherited predisposing factor or due the trophic effect of gastrin, or the lack of corpus atrophy.

Mechanisms of altered hormone release

There are two main theories to explain the altered gastric physiology (Figure 3.11). Firstly, ammonia from *H. pylori*'s urease [28] may be responsible. This might act directly through an effect of ammonia itself on endocrine cells, or by increasing the local pH [97]. More probably, ammonia reacts with hydrochloric acid in the presence of oxygen free radicals from neutrophils to produce monochloramine which increases both gastrin release and acid secretion in rats [108]. Secondly certain cytokines including tumour necrosis factor-alpha

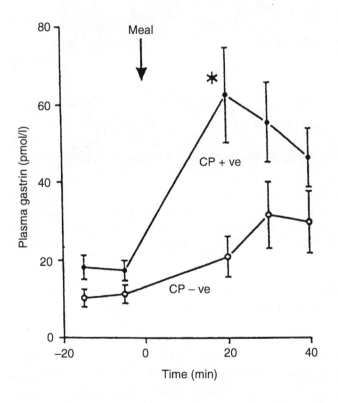

Figure 3.7 The demonstration by Levi *et al.* [97] that plasma gastrin concentrations are elevated in patients infected with *H. pylori*. It took 18 months to find six uninfected duodenal ulcer patients in our clinic! (*Source:* from reference 97, with permission.)

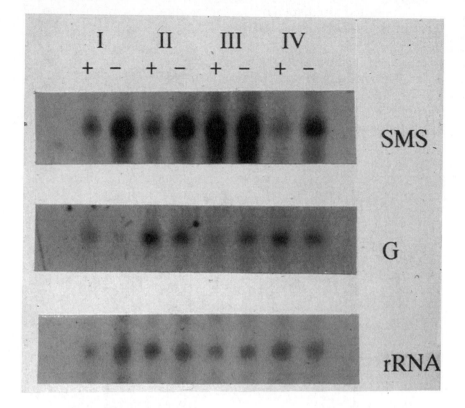

Figure 3.8 Northern blot showing antral somatostatin mRNA (SMS) in four patients, I–IV, before (+) and after (−) eradication of *H. pylori*. Probing for ribosomal RNA (rRNA) showed that a similar amount of RNA was loaded on to each lane. There was a significant rise in somatostatin mRNA after therapy. (*Source*: from reference 100, with permission.)

and interferon-gamma are able to release gastrin from endocrine cells *in vitro* and might be responsible [109,110].

Toxins
H. pylori can be divided into toxigenic and non-toxigenic strains. In general, toxigenic strains of *H. pylori* have the entire *vacA* gene and express its product, vacuolating toxin (87 kDa) [31]. They also possess and express the *cagA* gene [32] and have circulating antibodies to its product CagA (128 kDa). Patients with ulcers are infected with toxigenic strains significantly more often than non-ulcer patients [111,112], suggesting that the strain of *H. pylori* present is an important determinant of whether ulcers form or not. However, most

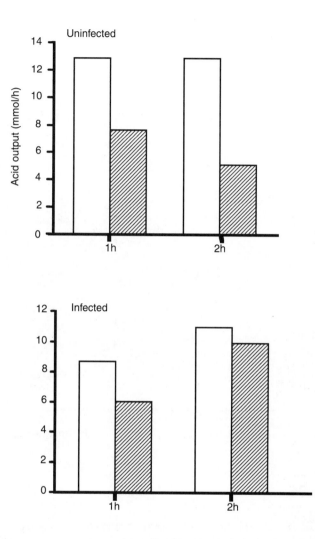

Figure 3.9 Peptone-stimulated acid secretion in volunteers with and without *H. pylori* infection, measured by intragastric titration. Open bars: pH 7.0; shaded bars: pH 2.5. Acid secretion is inhibited by the low pH, particularly in the second hour in uninfected subjects, but acid secretion is not inhibited at this time in infected subjects. (*Source*: drawn from data in reference 106.)

workers have measured antibodies rather than the toxin itself. In that case the results reflect the strength of the patient's immune response as well as whether or not the bacteria produces toxin.

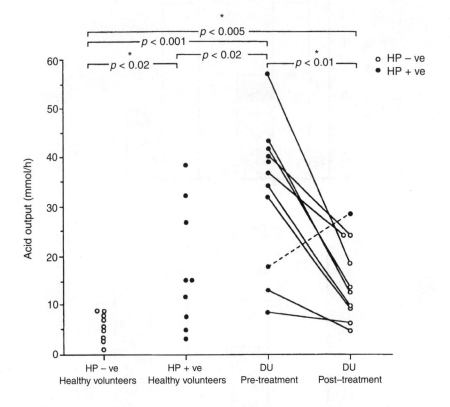

Figure 3.10 Acid secretion stimulated by infusions of gastrin-releasing peptide (GRP) in different groups of individuals. GRP-stimulated acid secretion is elevated in infected volunteers and even more so in patients with duodenal ulcers (DU). Treatment of *H. pylori* infection leads to a fall in GRP-stimulated acid secretion. (*Source*: from reference 107, with permission.)

Gastric metaplasia in the duodenum

This phenomenon, which allows *H. pylori* to colonize the duodenum, may play a major role in allowing the bacteria to cause local damage in that region. It probably results from repeated injury to the duodenum by acid and is discussed in more detail above.

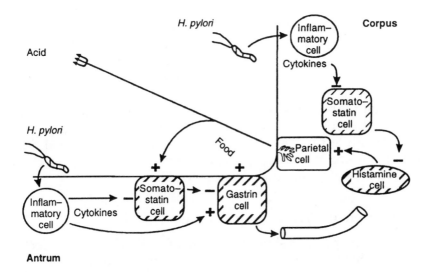

Figure 3.11 Schematic diagram of gastric physiology in *H. pylori* infection. Food stimulates acid secretion through release of histamine and gastrin. This system is restrained by local release of the inhibitory peptide somatostatin. It is envisaged that inflammatory cytokines inhibit somatostatin release and increase release of gastrin. Products of *H. pylori* itself may also be involved (see text).

CHRONIC GASTRIC ULCERS

Introduction

A gastric ulcer is a breach in the gastric epithelium. This section describes chronic gastric ulcers, rather than the acute ulcers frequently seen in severely ill patients with major trauma, head injuries, burns and sepsis.

Epidemiology

Chronic gastric ulcers (GUs) are quite common. At any time about 0.3% of the Finnish population has one [67]. The lifetime prevalence of GUs is 4% in males and 3% in females [68]. About 0.02% of the population develops a GU for the first time in any year [113]. The prevalence of GUs is similar in males and females. They are rare under the age of 40 years and tend to occur in the lower socioeconomic groups [68]. Reported infection rates in patients with GUs vary from 58–94% [79,114]. It is difficult to attribute this range of rates to geographical differences because both the lowest and the highest prevalences are reported from Finland. One problem is that GU patients tend to have extensive gastric atrophy. This can produce false-negative biopsy-based tests because the patches of intestinal metaplasia in the stomach are not infected. Therefore it is wise to take multiple biopsies for examination. It is also advisable to test GU patients for infection using other methods such as serology or the urea breath test before accepting that they are not infected. Most genuinely uninfected GU patients are taking NSAIDs, which are presumably the cause of their ulcers [115].

H. pylori eradication in the management of GUs

Gastric ulcer patients should be treated for *H. pylori* if this infection is found. Studies have consistently shown that recurrence of gastric ulcers is greatly diminished by therapy that aims to eradicate the bacterium. Graham *et al.* reported 2-year relapse rates of 13% after ranitidine plus triple therapy, compared with 74% in patients given ranitidine alone [115] (Figure 3.12). Both the two patients whose ulcers recurred after the eradication regimen had persistent infection and were taking NSAIDs. Karita *et al.* reported a 1-year GU relapse rate of 0% after successful eradication, compared with 75% in those with persisting infection [116].

It seems worthwhile to use an eradication regimen at the start of treatment for a GU. Labenz and Borsch found that GUs heal more rapidly if the regimen eradicates the infection. The rate of ulcer healing at 6 weeks was 85% if the bacterium was eventually eradicated, compared with 60% if it was not [117]. This does not strictly prove that eradication accelerates healing, because a failure to eradicate could reflect a factor, such as poor compliance or high acid secretion, decreasing healing and eradication independently. However there seems no good reason to delay eradication therapy, particularly as eradication of *H. pylori* has been found to be effective in healing GUs (and DUs) that are resistant to other forms of therapy [118]. Eradication of *H. pylori* greatly diminishes the risk of subsequent haemorrhage in patients who have bled from a GU. None of the GU patients treated by Labenz and Borsch rebled during a median follow-up of 17 months if *H. pylori* had been successfully eradicated, compared with 36% of those with persisting infection [84].

The clinical management of GUs is discussed in Chapter 6. Strategy is dominated by the malignant potential of GUs. *H. pylori* infection is now recognized to be a carcinogen so it seems sensible to eradicate it from patients with GUs who are at risk of cancer. However there is currently no evidence that eradication of long-standing *H. pylori* infection alters the risk of cancer in GU patients or, for that matter, in any other group of individuals.

Aetiological theories

It is now quite clear that *H. pylori* is an important aetiological factor in GU disease because recurrence is prevented by eradication of this infection [115,116]. However, other factors must be important because not everybody who is infected develops a GU.

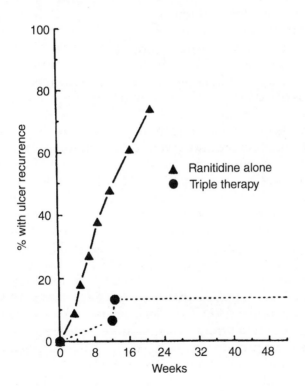

Figure 3.12 Recurrence of gastric ulcers after treatment with either ranitidine alone or ranitidine plus an *H. pylori* eradication regimen. (*Source:* from reference 115, with permission.)

Ulcers occur when luminal aggressive factors overcome mucosal defence. As regards the former, acid clearly plays some role in GU disease because ulcer healing is faster and recurrences are less likely when acid secretion is suppressed [119]. However acid cannot be regarded as a primary cause of GUs because these patients secrete, on average, less acid and pepsin than controls [120]. Indeed, GUs occur occasionally in patients with no measurable acid secretion at all [121]. Refluxed duodenal contents might be important in GU disease because these patients have more duodeno-gastric reflux than controls. In one study reflux occurred in 81% of GU patients compared with 42% of controls [122]. This exposes the gastric mucosa to injurious agents in duodenal juice, including pancreatic enzymes, bile salts and lysolecithin [47]. However duodeno-gastric reflux is not universally present in GU disease so it seems likely that ulceration is mainly due to a weakness of the gastric mucosa.

Several factors are thought to weaken the mucosa. Gastric ulcers tend to occur in an epithelium which is affected by chronic gastritis with atrophy and intestinal metaplasia [123]. This is why these patients secrete less acid [120]. The changes seen on histology are probably caused by chronic *H. pylori* infection interacting with other factors such as duodeno-gastric reflux and the patient's class II type, as discussed above. Chronic gastritis in GU patients is likely to decrease mucosal resistance in a number of ways. For example, normal gastric mucosa produces pancreatic secretory trypsin inhibitor which inhibits refluxed pancreatic enzymes, but less of this is present in the mucosa of GU patients [124]. Gastritis is a diffuse process, so why do GUs occur at particular sites? They have been found to occur at the junction between antral and corpus mucosa, or at the junction between normal and metaplastic epithelium. These junctional regions may be particularly unstable [125].

GUs usually occur on the lesser curve of the stomach. Several theories have been proposed to explain this. The antral mucosa often extends up the lesser curve, so that this part of the stomach presents an extensive junctional region. The lesser curve may also be particularly subject to trauma from ingested food. In addition the lesser curve may be more prone to ischaemia because it is supplied by end arteries, unlike the remainder of the stomach [126].

H. pylori may cause GUs by producing chronic gastritis over many years but eradication of this infection has a rapid effect on the rate of ulcer recurrence [115,116]. This indicates that an immediate effect of factors released by *H. pylori* itself or by the leucocytes that it attracts is also important in the production of ulcers.

H. pylori, gastric ulcers and NSAIDs

We have been slower to establish the role of *H. pylori* in GU disease than in DU disease. One factor which complicates research is that GUs have another important cause, namely NSAIDs. NSAIDs cause GUs more often than they cause DUs [127]. It seems likely that most of the GUs that occur in uninfected patients are due to NSAID therapy. Graham found that his GU patients who were not infected with *H. pylori* had NSAIDs or their metabolites detectable in their blood or urine.

An important clinical point is whether it is worth eradicating *H. pylori*, if it is present, from a patient who has developed dyspepsia while taking NSAIDs. In practice it seems sensible to do so but the scientific basis for this is less clear. *H. pylori* and NSAIDs both independently cause dyspepsia, ulcers and ulcer complications, but it is not clear whether such problems are more prevalent in patients who are both infected and take NSAIDs. Data on this are conflicting. Several studies have asked whether the prevalence of *H. pylori* infection is altered in individuals who are taking NSAIDs. The general conclusion is that it is not [128], but some studies have shown *less* infection in NSAID takers [129,130]. This has even led to the suggestion that NSAIDs have an antibacterial effect [130], but other explanations seem more likely. Patients with *H. pylori* may have ulcers more often and may therefore avoid taking NSAIDs. Two studies showed that infected persons are more likely to develop dyspepsia when they take NSAIDs and therefore to stop taking them than uninfected persons [131,132], but this tendency has not been found by some other groups [132]. Another question is whether endoscopic gastritis is greater if NSAIDs are taken by a person who is infected with *H. pylori*. The general conclusion is that it is not [128,132–134]. Curiously, Graham *et al.* found **less** [128] but Hudson *et al.* found **more** [135] haemorrhagic lesions in persons who were infected with *H. pylori* and took NSAIDs.

Does *H. pylori* infection make an NSAID-taker more likely to develop a GU? Apparently so, although the data is relatively scanty. Two studies have shown that gastric ulcers are more prevalent in patients afflicted by both NSAIDs and *H. pylori* than in patients who have only one of these adverse factors [135,136]. Being infected increased the risk of developing an ulcer during NSAID therapy by about twofold. A third study gave a similar results and highlighted the role of gastritis in the risk of developing a GU. Reactive (or chemical) gastritis was first described in patients with duodeno-gastric reflux following gastric surgery by Dixon [137] and is also seen in a proportion of patients who take NSAIDs [138]. It consists of foveolar hyperplasia, vasodilation, oedema and a paucity of inflammatory cells. Taha *et al.* [138] found reactive gastritis in 26% of patients who had taken NSAIDs for at least 4 weeks. Ulcers were found in 48% of patients with *H. pylori* gastritis and 54% of patients with reactive gastritis compared with only 22% of patients who were taking NSAIDs but had neither form of gastritis. Overall the patients taking NSAIDs were more likely to have a GU (or a DU) if they were infected with *H. pylori*. Therefore we have the evidence that *H. pylori* infection increases the risk of developing an ulcer while taking NSAIDs. However, despite this, preliminary evidence suggests that *H. pylori* eradication does not influence healing or ulcer recurrence in NSAID-related ulcers.

More work is required, but at present, despite the contradiction, it seems worthwhile eradicating *H. pylori* from a patient who is infected and develops an ulcer while taking NSAIDs. After all it might be the infection, rather than the drug, that is causing the ulcer in that particular patient.

NON-ULCER DYSPEPSIA

Introduction

It is marvellous that eradication of *H. pylori* can cure duodenal and gastric ulcers, but most dyspepsia is not due to these. The relationship between *H. pylori* and non-ulcer dyspepsia (NUD) is of crucial importance in the design of clinical strategies (Chapter 6). Does *H. pylori* causes NUD or not? First we need to define NUD. Bianchi Porro and Parente have recently written an excellent review of this topic [139].

The nature of non-ulcer dyspepsia

There is still no generally agreed definition of what dyspepsia is. The term means 'bad digestion' so symptoms are presumed to emanate from the upper gastrointestinal tract. Thompson introduced the term 'non-ulcer dyspepsia' (NUD) in 1984 to denote 'a chronic, recurrent, often meal-related epigastric discomfort initially suspected to be due a peptic ulcer but not subsequently found to be so' [140]. The term has become internationally accepted to indicate patients with persistent upper gastrointestinal symptoms for more than 1

month in the absence of gastrointestinal or systemic disease [141].
In 1984 Lagarde and Spiro also proposed the term 'functional
dyspepsia', which has the same meaning [142].

Prevalence

It has been estimated that as many as 20–30% of Western populations have NUD but these data are questionable, not least because
of the lack of a clear definition of the condition. For example a large
study in Minnesota gave a figure of 26%, but almost a third of these
had a history of peptic ulcer disease. NUD appears to be commoner
under the age of 25 years but is also found in the elderly, suggesting
that it is a lifelong condition. In one study two-thirds of patients still
had symptoms after 5 years, although in most patients the symptoms were not sufficiently severe to interfere with their ability to
work.

Subgroups of NUD

One view is that NUD actually comprises a number of subgroups,
which present with different symptoms, have different aetiologies
and require different investigations and treatment. These are:

- **ulcer-like dyspepsia**: these patients have classical ulcer symptoms, but no ulcer;
- **dysmotility-like dyspepsia**: patients whose dyspeptic symptoms suggest gastric stasis or dysmotility of the small-bowel;
- **reflux-like dyspepsia**: in these patients dyspepsia includes
  symptoms suggestive of gastro-oesophageal reflux;
- **unspecified dyspepsia**: this term is reserved for dyspeptics who
  do not fall into any of the above groups!

Most clinicians will recognize these patterns, but this classification is not proving particularly useful in research because many
patients fall into more than one subgroup [143] and the symptom
clusters do not predict the patient's physiological disorder [144].

NUD and gastro-oesophageal reflux

Gastro-oesophageal reflux (GOR) is probably the commonest reason
for chronic antacid ingestion [145]. It typically presents with heart-
burn and regurgitation of acid into the mouth, but over a third of
patients also have symptoms referable to the upper abdomen such

as epigastric pain, nausea or vomiting, so that it is often difficult to differentiate between NUD and GOR on the basis of symptoms alone. About 20% of patients with endoscopy negative NUD were found to have GOR on detailed work-up including oesophageal pH monitoring [144]. GOR and NUD might occur together by coincidence, but it seems most likely that the two sets of symptoms are caused by the same disturbance.

NUD and irritable bowel syndrome

The irritable bowel syndrome (IBS) is the commonest gastrointestinal disease and presents with abdominal discomfort and a disorder of bowel habit. Abdominal pain occurs in both IBS and NUD but the former is diagnosed if the pain is related to defecation [146,147]. As many as 30% of dyspeptics also have IBS [148]. According to Sielaff these complain of food intolerance, belching and nausea more often than patients with NUD alone [149], but Talley *et al.* [148] found that patients with IBS do not fall into any particular subgroup of dyspepsia. Again, NUD might occur with IBS by coincidence but it seems more likely that there is a common underlying disturbance.

Non-ulcer dyspepsia and *H. pylori* infection

At present we do not know whether *H. pylori* causes NUD or not. This is frustrating because NUD is such a common condition. Researchers have attempted to explore the relationship by asking the following questions:

Are NUD patients infected more often than controls?
Dyspepsia was commoner in seropositive *versus* seronegative blood donors, but these results do not help because the subjects were not endoscoped to see if they had ulcers. Four endoscopic surveys showed *H. pylori* infection in 43–79% of NUD patients. These numbers were well above control in three of these surveys, but the results are inconclusive because the controls were not properly matched for age [150,151]. In short it seems likely that *H. pylori* is more prevalent in patients with NUD, but better studies are needed.

Is H. pylori more prevalent in any specific subgroup of NUD?
Acute *H. pylori* causes dyspeptic symptoms (see above) [8,152]. Whether chronic *H. pylori* infection causes symptoms is less clear,

particularly as at least 50% of infected persons have no symptoms [153]. Some have found that infected persons are more likely to have ulcer-like [154] or reflux-like symptoms [150]. However most surveys have not shown an association between chronic *H. pylori* infection and any particular symptom complex [155,156].

Does eradication of H. pylori relieve symptoms of NUD?
This seems the obvious approach, but there are problems.

* There has been no standard way to measure dyspepsia.
* It is difficult to do double-blind studies with bismuth because it discolours the stools.
* Drugs such as bismuth and omeprazole may improve dyspepsia, independently of their effect on *H. pylori*.

Initial studies asked whether dyspeptic symptoms were better when the patients took bismuth than when they took placebo. The general conclusion of these trials was that bismuth improves dyspepsia but that this has nothing to do with whether *H. pylori* is suppressed or not [157]. Similarly, Patchett *et al.* [158] saw an improvement during therapy with bismuth, with or without antibiotics, and this was independent of whether *H. pylori* was eradicated. Their follow-up period was 6–12 months, which should allowed time for bismuth to leave the body. McCarthy *et al.* have used omeprazole-based regimen and followed patients for 12 months. Eradication did improve dyspepsia, but the effect was only significant during the second 6-month period [159]. This is very encouraging, but the study was not strictly double blind, so there could have been a 'placebo' effect. Therefore we still lack unequivocal evidence that eradication of *H. pylori* improves NUD.

H. pylori infection and gastroduodenal motility

Several groups have asked whether the abnormal gastroduodenal motility which is present in about 60% of NUD patients [160,161] is due to *H. pylori*, but there is no good evidence that this is the case. Wegener *et al.* [162] reported that patients with *H. pylori* infection have delayed gastric emptying, but three other studies, for example that of Tucci *et al.* [154], failed to confirm this. Pieramico, Ditschuneit and Malfertheiner [163] found that antral motility was abnormal in patients with NUD whether they were infected or not.

Principles of management of NUD

There is no general consensus on the treatment of NUD, but division of patients into the four classical clusters may be helpful. Suppression of acid secretion appears to be most helpful in 'reflux-like' and 'ulcer-like' dyspepsias. Prokinetic agents are of most use in 'dysmotility-like' and 'reflux-like' dyspepsias. 'Indeterminate dyspepsia' is least understood so either approach may be tried.

The role of eradicating *H. pylori* remains unclear but preliminary data suggest that this may be most helpful in 'ulcer-like' dyspepsia. Eradication rates may be higher in NUD patients than in DU patients, perhaps because of their lower rates of acid secretion.

SPECIFIC FORMS OF GASTROPATHY

H. pylori and Ménétrier's disease

Patients with Ménétrier's disease have giant gastric folds and foveolar hyperplasia. The amount of mucosal inflammation is variable. The role of *H. pylori* remains unclear. Two studies found low rates of infection in Ménétrier's disease [164,165], but another saw *H. pylori* on histology in 88% of 138 patients [166]. The degree of gastritis was greater in the infected patients. Furthermore, eradication of *H. pylori* from a 28-year-old woman produced a marked improvement in mucosal histology and a decrease in protein loss [167].

H. pylori and congestive gastropathy

Congestive gastropathy is a term used to describe the congested stomach found in patients with portal hypertension and gastric varices. Two studies showed low rates of infection in this condition [168,169].

GASTRIC CANCER

Introduction

Clinicians should worry more about asymptomatic *H. pylori* infection if they know that it increases the risk of gastric cancer. This is now established, and in 1994 the World Health Organization added *H. pylori* to its list of known carcinogens. Proving the causal relationship has been more difficult for cancer than for ulcers. One problem for researchers is that it takes decades for the infection to cause cancer, so it is difficult to test whether eradication decreases the incidence of cancer. The other problem is that gastric atrophy, a step in the carcinogenic process, may decrease or even eliminate the infection by the time the tumour develops. The idea that *H. pylori* causes gastric cancer comes firstly from evidence that this infection initiates histological processes associated with gastric cancer. Secondly, studies show that people with *H. pylori* infection are more likely to develop gastric cancer. In both sorts of studies it has been necessary to ask whether *H. pylori* might be an 'innocent bystander' but, taken overall, the evidence is already convincing.

Epidemiology

Gastric cancer is clearly an important disease. In the United Kingdom 12 300 people developed gastric cancer in 1985 (Cancer Research Campaign factsheet) and gastric cancer represented 6% of all cancers. Worldwide in 1985 it affected 10 million persons, which makes it the second most prevalent cancer behind lung cancer (12 million) [170]. Gastric cancer occurs much more frequently in developing countries than in developed countries, where the incidence of gastric cancer is falling quite rapidly. This decrease started earliest in countries with well-developed economies such as the USA and Northern Europe [171] (Figure 3.13). In the UK, Barker showed that gastric cancer prevalence in different regions in 1968–78 correlated strongly with overcrowding in that particular region in 1936 [172]. In people who moved from one region of the country to another the incidence of cancer correlated with their place of birth rather than where they ended up, suggesting that the early environment is important.

Geographical relationships between H. pylori and gastric cancer
Studies within countries have given conflicting results. Studies in Colombia [173] and China [174] showed higher prevalence in regions with high cancer risk, but studies in Italy [175] and Costa Rica [176] did not. Interestingly in China the regional prevalence of cancer incidence only correlated with the prevalence of *H. pylori* in children under 5 years old, consistent with the view that early infection has the greatest effect [174].

The Eurogast study showed a positive correlation between the prevalences of gastric cancer and *H. pylori* in different countries around the world [177]. The correlation was convincing and statistically significant. If one accepts that childhood infection causes cancer in later life, some of the variability in the results might be due to changes in national prevalences of *H. pylori* since the current cancer patients were children. The scatter of results might also reflect the role of other factors, such as diet. There is good evidence that diets high in salt, nitrates and preserved food predispose to gastric cancer, while diets high in fruit and vegetables protect [178].

The relationship between H. pylori infection and gastric cancer in individuals

Initial studies examined the prevalence of infection in individuals who had already developed cancer. The results were conflicting, with odds ratios ranging from 0.5–4.2. However, this might have been because infection that was previously present was either undetectable or absent by the time the cancer had been diagnosed [178].

Therefore more recent studies have looked 'prospectively' at the fate of people with stored serum available from years ago. Testing of these stored sera shows a clear association between infection and subsequent cancer [179–181]. The odds ratio is greatest in the studies with the oldest sera [178]. Thus the matched odds ratio rises from 2.1, in studies with sera collected less than 5 years ago, progressively to 8.7 in patients known to be infected ≥ 15 years ago [178].

'H. pylori causes gastritis, which causes cancer'

H. pylori is also implicated in gastric carcinogenesis by its role in the progression which is generally regarded as leading to this gastric cancer. Early gastric cancers develop in areas of intestinal metaplasia or chronic atrophic gastritis [182]. Correa pioneered the idea that gastric cancer develops through a progression of gastritis via atrophy to metaplasia then to dysplasia before cancer [183]. This idea was supported by longitudinal studies, for example in Finland [184]. *H. pylori* is implicated because it is the commonest cause of gastritis [79]. Also, we now know that atrophic gastritis, which was previously regarded as more or less part of the normal ageing process, actually occurs selectively in persons infected with *H. pylori* [48]. *H. pylori* is epidemiologically associated with the intestinal but not with the diffuse type of gastric cancer [185]. This supports the idea that the development of intestinal metaplasia is an important step in the chain of events that leads from asymptomatic infection to gastric cancer.

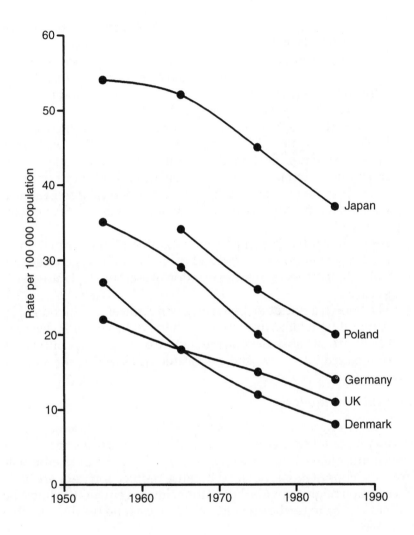

Figure 3.13 Falling incidence of gastric cancer deaths in different countries. Comparison with Figure 2.1 shows that the prevalence of cancer is related to the national prevalence of *H. pylori* in older persons. (*Source*: drawn from data in Kurihara, Aoki, Hismaichi, eds. *Cancer mortality statistics in the world*. Nagoya: University of Nagoya Press, 1989.)

Possible carcinogenic mechanisms

There are a number of interesting ideas. Briefly, these are as follows.

- *H. pylori* causes gastric atrophy, which elevates the intragastric pH [48]. The lack of acid allows the growth of nitrate-reducing bacteria (not *H. pylori*), which produce nitrite, which is in turn converted to carcinogenic N-nitroso compounds [186]. Interestingly, a high salt diet also causes chronic gastritis and increases the incidence of gastric cancer [187].
- Prolonged inflammation of other organs tends to increase the likelihood of cancer. Examples include hepatitis B virus, human papilloma virus, Epstein–Barr virus and schistosomiasis. The mechanism remains open to speculation, but neutrophils attracted into the mucosa by *H. pylori* release oxygen free radicals which have been implicated in carcinogenesis in other organs [188].
- Ascorbic acid is an important inhibitor of the formation of N-nitroso compounds [186] and inactivator of oxygen free radicals. *H. pylori* decreases the secretion of ascorbic acid into gastric juice [38].
- The known association between gastric cancer and blood group A might be related in some way to the adhesion of *H. pylori* to blood-group substances on the surface of the gastric epithelium, or secreted into saliva and gastric juice [21].

Clinical consequences

There is strong evidence that *H. pylori* is a gastric carcinogen. Its elimination might prevent hundreds of thousands of gastric cancers in a country like China. However, *H. pylori* is difficult to eliminate from such populations, not least because re-infection rates are high. Vaccination might provide the solution. Improvements to sanitation will slowly decrease the prevalence of *H. pylori* and the diseases that it causes.

The implications for clinical practice in Western countries are less clear. In particular, as childhood infection seems important and it is not clear whether eradicating *H. pylori* from a middle-aged person will have any effect. This may depend on how reversible changes such as atrophy and intestinal metaplasia prove to be. It appears that atrophy can reverse [65], but more studies are needed.

From the practical point of view I would recommend eradicating *H. pylori* if it is found in a young person. I did so in myself at the age of 45 years. However, gastric cancer is disappearing from the Western world so rapidly that there is danger of it vanishing just as we learn to prevent it!

GASTRIC LYMPHOMA

Introduction

Lymphocytes are more or less absent from uninfected gastric mucosa, but universally present when the mucosa is infected with *H. pylori*. This has led researchers to ask whether this infection predisposes to the development of gastric lymphomas. The evidence indicates that this is the case and, remarkably, that some tumours regress when *H. pylori* is eradicated.

Gastric MALT lymphomas

Isaacson, of University College London, has studied the immune system of the gut and developed the concept of mucosa-associated lymphoid tissue (MALT) [189]. The lymphocytes found in *H. pylori*-infected gastric mucosa constitute an example of acquired MALT – as opposed to Peyer's patches, which are normally present. It has been suggested that lymphoid follicles are to be found in all infected persons if sufficient biopsies are examined [43]. They are collections of B-cells. Wotherspoon *et al.* studied 450 patients with *H. pylori* gastritis and found lymphoid follicles in 125 [190]. B-cells infiltrated the epithelium in 8 cases (Figure 3.20). The lesion is then called a MALT lymphoma, although it remains debatable whether it is strictly a neoplasm. Wotherspoon *et al.* found that *H. pylori* was present in 101 out of 110 patients with gastric MALT lymphoma (92%) [190]. Furthermore, and remarkably, eradication of *H. pylori* led to disappearance of low-grade MALT lymphomas in five out of six patients [45]. This finding has since been confirmed by others.

Primary gastric non-Hodgkin's lymphoma

The stomach is the commonest site of extranodal lymphomas. These tumours constitute 3% of all gastric neoplasms and 10% of all lymphomas. Parsonnet *et al.* asked whether *H. pylori* infection increases the risk of gastric non-Hodgkin's lymphoma. Their results show that patients with this type of tumour are indeed six times more likely to be infected with *H. pylori* than controls. They estimate that 60% of these tumours are attributable to *H. pylori* infection [41].

Clinical implications

These findings provide another argument for eradicating *H. pylori* from asymptomatic persons. In patients with gastric lymphomas it is worth diagnosing and curing *H. pylori* infection before considering more drastic therapies because there are several reports of tumour regression. There are even reports of non-Hodgkin's lymphomas shrinking, but more research is needed.

The possible role of *H. pylori* in vascular disease is discussed in Chapter 7.

REFERENCES

1. Dixon MF. Histological responses to *H. pylori* infection: gastritis, atrophy and preneoplasia. In: Calam J, ed. Baillière's *Clinical Gastroenterology: Helicobacter pylori*. London: Baillière Tindall, 1995: **9**: 467–486.
2. Marshall BJ. *Campylobacter pyloridis* and gastritis. *J Infect Dis* 1986; **153**: 650–657.
3. Graham DY, Go MF, Evans DJJ. Review article: urease, gastric ammonium/ammonia, and *Helicobacter pylori* – the past, the present, and recommendations for future research. *Aliment Pharmacol Ther* 1992; **6**: 659–669.
4. Marshall BJ. Virulence and pathogenicity of *Helicobacter pylori*. *J Gastroenterol Hepatol* 1991; **6**: 121–124.
5. Denizot Y, Sobhani I, Rambaud JC *et al*. Paf-acether synthesis by *Helicobacter pylori*. *Gut* 1990; **31**: 1242–1245.
6. Crabtree JE, Peichl P, Wyatt JI *et al*. Gastric interleukin-8 and IgA IL-8 autoantibodies in *Helicobacter pylori* infection. *Scand J Immunol* 1993; **37**: 65–70.
7. Morris AJ, Ali MR, Nicholson GI *et al*. Long-term follow-up of voluntary ingestion of *Helicobacter pylori*. *Ann Intern Med* 1991; **114**: 662–663.
8. Ramsey EJ, Carey KV, Peterson WL *et al*. Epidemic gastritis with hypochlorhydria. *Gastroenterology* 1979; **76**: 1449–1457.
9. Graham DY, Alpert LC, Smith JL, Yoshimura HH. Iatrogenic *Campylobacter pylori* infection is a cause of epidemic achlorhydria. *Am J Gastroenterol* 1988; **83**: 974–980.

10. Cave DR, Vargas M. Effect of a *Campylobacter pylori* protein on acid secretion by parietal cells. *Lancet* 1989; **ii**: 187–189.
11. Noach LA, Bosma NB *et al*. Mucosal tumor necrosis factor-alpha, interleukin-1 beta, and interleukin-8 production in patients with *Helicobacter pylori* infection. *Scand J Gastroenterol* 1994; **29**: 425–429.
12. Tache Y, Saperas E. Potent inhibition of gastric acid secretion and ulcer formation by centrally and peripherally administered interleukin-1. *Ann N Y Acad Sci* 1992; **664**: 353–368.
13. Hunt RH. *Campylobacter pylori* and spontaneous hypochlorhydria. In: Rathbone BJ, Heatley RV, eds. *Campylobacter pylori and gastroduodenal disease*. London: Blackwell, 1989: 176–184.
14. Axon ATR. Acute infection with *H. pylori*. In: Hunt RH, Tytgat GNJ, eds. *Helicobacter pylori: Basic mechanisms to clinical cure*. Lancaster: Kluwer Academic Publications, 1994: 407–412.
15. Wiersinga WM, Tytgat GN. Clinical recovery owing to target parietal cell failure in a patient with Zollinger–Ellison syndrome. *Gastroenterology* 1977; **73**: 1413–1417.
16. Faber K. Chronic gastritis in relation to achylia and ulcer. *Lancet* 1927; **i**: 901.
17. Strickland RG, Mackay IR. A reappraisal of the nature and significance of chronic atrophic gastritis. *Am J Dig Dis* 1973; **18**: 426–440.
18. Glass GBJ, Pitchumoni CS. Atrophic gastritis. *Hum Pathol* 1975; **6**: 219–250.
19. Misiewicz JJ, Tytgat GNJ, Goodwin CS. The Sydney system: a new classification of gastritis. *J Hepatol Gastroenterol* 1991; **6**: 209–222.
20. Hessey SJ, Spencer J, Wyatt JI *et al*. Bacterial adhesion and disease activity in *Helicobacter* associated chronic gastritis. *Gut* 1990; **31**: 134–138.
21. Boren T, Falk P, Roth KA *et al*. Attachment of *Helicobacter pylori* to human gastric epithelium mediated by blood group antigens. *Science* 1993; **262**: 1892–1895.
22. Sobala GM, Wyatt JI, Dixon MF. Histological aspects of atrophic gastritis. In: Holt PR, Russell RM, eds. *Chronic gastritis and hypochlorhydria in the elderly*. Boca Raton, FL: CRC Press, 1993: 49–68.
23. Bayerdorffer E, Lehn N, Hatz R *et al*. Difference in expression of *Helicobacter pylori* gastritis in antrum and body. *Gastroenterology* 1992; **102**: 1575–1582.

24. Graham DY, Go MF. *Helicobacter pylori*: current status. *Gastroenterology* 1993; **105**: 279–282.
25. Blaser MJ. Hypotheses on the pathogenesis and natural history of *Helicobacter pylori*-induced inflammation. *Gastroenterology* 1992; **102**: 720–727.
26. Christensen AH, Gjorup T, Hilden J *et al*. Observer homogeneity in the histologic diagnosis of *Helicobacter pylori*. Latent class analysis, kappa coefficient, and repeat frequency. *Scand J Gastroenterol* 1992; **27**: 933–939.
27. Crabtree J, Wyatt J. Host responses. In: Northfield TC, Mendall M, Goggin PM, eds. *Helicobacter pylori infection*. Lancaster: Kluwer Academic Publishers, 1993: 40–52.
28. Hu LT, Mobley HL. Expression of catalytically active recombinant *Helicobacter pylori* urease at wild-type levels in *Escherichia coli*. *Infect Immun* 1993; **61**: 2563–2569.
29. Nielsen H, Birkholz S, Andersen LP, Moran AP. Neutrophil activation by *Helicobacter pylori* lipopolysaccharides. *J Infect Dis* 1994; **170**: 135–139.
30. Dunn BE, Roop RM, Sung CC *et al*. Identification and purification of a cpn60 heat shock protein homolog from *Helicobacter pylori*. *Infect Immun* 1992; **60**: 1946–1951.
31. Cover TL, Blaser MJ. Purification and characterization of the vacuolating toxin from *Helicobacter pylori*. *J Biol Chem* 1992; **267**: 10570–10575.
32. Tummuru MK, Cover TL, Blaser MJ. Cloning and expression of a high-molecular-mass major antigen of *Helicobacter pylori*: evidence of linkage to cytotoxin production. *Infect Immun* 1993; **61**: 1799–1809.
33. Crabtree JE, Shallcross TM, Heatley RV, Wyatt JI. Mucosal tumour necrosis factor alpha and interleukin-6 in patients with *Helicobacter pylori* associated gastritis. Gut 1991; **32**: 1473–1477.
34. Wee A, Teh M, Raju GC. Expression of HLA-DR antigen in different histological types of gastric polyp. *J Clin Pathol* 1992; **45**: 509–512.
35. Beales ILP, Davey N, Scunes D *et al*. HLA Class II type and *H. pylori*-induced gastric atrophy (abstract). *Gut* 1994; **35**(suppl 5): S45.
36. Azuma T, Konishi J, Tanaka Y *et al*. Contribution of HLA-DQA gene to host's response against *Helicobacter pylori* (letter). *Lancet* 1994; **343**: 542–543.
37. Davies GR, Simmonds NJ, Stevens TR *et al*. Mucosal reactive

oxygen metabolite production in duodenal ulcer disease. *Gut* 1992; **33**: 1467–1472.

38. Sobala GM, Schorah CJ, Shires S *et al.* Effect of eradication of *Helicobacter pylori* on gastric juice ascorbic acid concentrations. *Gut* 1993; **34**: 1038–1041.

39. Phull PS, Gower JD, Price AB *et al.* α-Tocopherol (vitamin E) antioxidant levels in chronic gastritis: correlation with mucosal neutrophil infiltration (abstract). *Gut* 1993; **34**(suppl 1): S34.

40. Hansson LE, Nyren O, Bergstrom R *et al.* Nutrients and gastric cancer risk. A population-based case-control study in Sweden. *Int J Cancer* 1994; **57**: 638–644.

41. Parsonnet J, Hansen S, Rodriguez L *et al. Helicobacter pylori* infection and gastric lymphoma. *N Engl J Med* 1994; **330**: 1267–1271.

42. Eidt S, Stolte M. Prevalence of lymphoid follicles and aggregates in *Helicobacter pylori* gastritis in antral and body mucosa. *J Clin Pathol* 1993; **46**: 832–835.

43. Genta RM, Hamner HW, Graham DY. Gastric lymphoid follicles in *Helicobacter pylori* infection: frequency, distribution, and response to triple therapy. *Hum Pathol* 1993; **24**: 577–583.

44. Rosh JR, Kurfist LA, Benkov KJ *et al. Helicobacter pylori* and gastric lymphonodular hyperplasia in children. *Am J Gastroenterol* 1992; **87**: 135–139.

45. Wotherspoon AC, Doglioni C, Diss TC *et al.* Regression of primary low-grade B-cell gastric lymphoma of mucosa-associated lymphoid tissue type after eradication of *Helicobacter pylori. Lancet* 1993; **342**: 575–577.

46. Wright NA, Pike C, Elia G. Induction of a novel epidermal growth factor-secreting cell lineage by mucosal ulceration in human gastrointestinal stem cells. *Nature* 1990; **343**: 82–85.

47. Sarosiek J, Slomiany BL, Slomiany A, Gabryelewicz A. Lysolecithin and glyceroglucolipids in gastric secretion of patients with gastric and duodenal ulcer. *Scand J Gastroenterol* 1983; **18**: 935–938.

48. Kuipers EJ, van Uffelen CWJ, Pals G *et al. Helicobacter pylori* and gastric mucosal atrophy (abstract). *Am J Gastroenterol* 1994; **89**: 1307.

49. Neithercut WD, Greig MA, Hossack M, McColl KE. Suicidal destruction of *Helicobacter pylori*: metabolic consequence of intracellular accumulation of ammonia. *J Clin Pathol* 1991; **44**: 380–384.

50. Karnes WE Jr, Samloff IM, Siurala M *et al.* Positive serum

antibody and negative tissue staining for *Helicobacter pylori* in subjects with atrophic body gastritis. *Gastroenterology* 1991; **101**: 167–174.

51. Negrini R, Lisato L, Zanella I *et al. Helicobacter pylori* infection induces antibodies cross-reacting with human gastric mucosa. *Gastroenterology* 1991; **101**: 437–445.

52. Andersen LP, Gaarslev K. IgG subclass antibodies against *Helicobacter pylori* heat-stable antigens in normal persons and in dyspeptic patients. *APMIS* 1992; **100**: 747–751.

53. Mathialagan R, Loizou S, Beales ILP *et al.* Who gets false-negative *H. pylori* (HP) ELISA results? (abstract). *Gut* 1994; **35**(suppl 5): S1.

54. Hermaszewski RA, Webster AD. Primary hypogamma-globulinaemia: a survey of clinical manifestations and complications. *Q J Med* 1993; **86**: 31–42.

55. Craanen ME, Blok P, Dekker W, Ferwerda J, Tytgat GN. Sub-types of intestinal metaplasia and *Helicobacter pylori*. *Gut* 1992; **33**: 597–600.

56. Sobala GM, O'Connor HJ, Dewar EP, King RF, Axon AT, Dixon MF. Bile reflux and intestinal metaplasia in gastric mucosa. *J Clin Pathol* 1993; **46**: 235–240.

57. Wyatt JI, Dixon MF. *Campylobacter*-associated chronic gastritis. *Pathol Annu* 1990; **25**: 75–98.

58. Sipponen P, Kekki M, Siurala M. The Sydney System: epide-miology and natural history of chronic gastritis. *J Gastroenterol Hepatol* 1991; **6**: 244–251.

59. Wyatt JI, Rathbone BJ, Sobala GM *et al.* Gastric epithelium in the duodenum: its association with *Helicobacter pylori* and inflammation. *J Clin Pathol* 1990; **43**: 981–986.

60. Tatsuta M, Iishi H, Yamamura H *et al.* Enhancement by tetragastrin of experimental induction of gastric epithelium in the duodenum. *Gut* 1989; **30**: 311–315.

61. Parrish JA, Rawlins DC. Intestinal mucosa in the Zollinger–Ellison syndrome. *Gut* 1965; **6**: 286–289.

62. Rhodes J, Evans KT, Lawrie JH, Forrest AP. Coarse mucosal folds in the duodenum. *Q J Med* 1968; **37**: 151–169.

63. Solcia E, Villani L, Fiocca R *et al.* Effects of eradication of *H. pylori* on gastritis in duodenal ulcer patients. *Scand J Gastroenterology* 1994; **29**(suppl 201): 28–34.

64. Wyatt JI, Rathbone BJ, Dixon MF, Heatley RV. *Campylobacter pyloridis* and acid induced gastric metaplasia in the pathogenesis of duodenitis. *J Clin Pathol* 1987; **40**: 841–848.

65. Borody TJ, Andrews P, Jankiewicz E *et al*. Apparent reversal of early gastric mucosal atrophy after triple therapy for *Helicobacter pylori*. *Am J Gastroenterol* 1993; **88**: 1266–1268.

66. Labenz J, Gyenes E, Ruhl GH *et al*. Is *Helicobacter pylori* gastritis a macroscopic diagnosis?. *Dtsch Med Wochenschr* 1993; **118**: 176–180.

67. Ihamaki T, Varis K, Siurala M. Morphological, functional and immunological state of the gastric mucosa in gastric carcinoma families. Comparison with a computer-matched family sample. *Scand J Gastroenterol* 1979; **14**: 801–812.

68. Langman MJS. *The epidemiology of chronic digestive disease.* London: Edward Arnold, 1979.

69. Bonnevie O. The incidence of duodenal ulcer in Copenhagen county. *Scand J Gastroenterol* 1975; **10**: 385–393.

70. Brinton W. *On the pathology, symptoms and treatment of ulcer of the stomach.* London: Churchill, 1867.

71. Susser S, Stein K. Civilisation and peptic ulcer. *Lancet* 1962; **i**: 115–118.

72. McCarthy DM. Smoking and ulcers – time to quit (editorial). *N Engl J Med* 1984; **311**: 726–728.

73. Somerville K, Faulkner G, Langman M. Non-steroidal anti-inflammatory drugs and bleeding peptic ulcer. *Lancet* 1986; **i**: 462–464.

74. Sonnenberg A, Muller Lissner SA, Vogel E *et al*. Predictors of duodenal ulcer healing and relapse. *Gastroenterology* 1981; **81**: 1061–1067.

75. Paffenbarger RS Jr, Wing AL, Hyde RT. Chronic disease in former college students: 13. Early precursors of peptic ulcer. *Am J Epidemiol* 1974; **100**: 307–315.

76. Malhotra SL. A comparison of unrefined wheat and rice diets in the management of duodenal ulcer. *Postgrad Med J* 1978; **54**: 6–9.

77. Gillberg R, Kastrup W, Mobacken H, Stockbrugger R, Ahren C. Gastric morphology and function in dermatitis herpetiformis and in coeliac disease. *Scand J Gastroenterol* 1985; **20**: 133–140.

78. Martin DF, Hollanders D, May SJ, Ravenscroft MM, Tweedle DE, Miller JP. Difference in relapse rates of duodenal ulcer after healing with cimetidine or tripotassium dicitrato bismuthate. *Lancet* 1981; **i**: 7–10.

79. Marshall BJ, Warren JR. Unidentified curved bacilli in the stomach of patients with gastritis and peptic ulceration. *Lancet* 1984; **i**: 1311–1315.

80. Marshall BJ, Goodwin CS, Warren JR *et al*. Prospective double-blind trial of duodenal ulcer relapse after eradication of *Campylobacter pylori*. *Lancet* 1988; **ii**: 1437–1442.

81. Rauws EA, Tytgat GN. Cure of duodenal ulcer associated with eradication of *Helicobacter pylori*. *Lancet* 1990; **335**: 1233–1235.

82. Tytgat G, Dixon M. Role in peptic ulcer disease: Overview. In: Northfield TC, Mendall M, Goggin PM, eds. *Helicobacter pylori infection*. Lancaster: Kluwer Academic Publishers, 1993: 75–87.

83. McColl KE, el Nujumi AM, Chittajallu RS *et al*. A study of the pathogenesis of *Helicobacter pylori* negative chronic duodenal ulceration. *Gut* 1993; **34**: 762–768.

84. Labenz J, Borsch G. Role of *Helicobacter pylori* eradication in the prevention of peptic ulcer bleeding relapse. *Digestion* 1994; **55**: 19–23.

85. Graham DY, Hepps KS, Ramirez FC *et al*. Treatment of *Helicobacter pylori* reduces the rate of rebleeding in peptic ulcer disease. *Scand J Gastroenterol* 1993; **28**: 939–942.

86. Reinbach DH, Cruickshank G, McColl KE. Acute perforated duodenal ulcer is not associated with *Helicobacter pylori* infection. *Gut* 1993; **34**: 1344–1347.

87. Rotter JI. The genetics of peptic ulcer: more than one gene, more than one disease. In: Steinberg AG, Bearn AG, Motulsky AG *et al*., eds. *Progress in Medical Genetics*. Philadelphia, PA: WB Saunders, 1980: 1–58.

88. Stewart DN, Winser DM. Incidence of perforated peptic ulcer: effect of heavy air-raids. *Lancet* 1942; **i**: 256–261.

89. Blair AJ, Feldman M, Barnett C *et al*. Detailed comparison of basal and food-stimulated gastric acid secretion rates and serum gastrin concentrations in duodenal ulcer patients and normal subjects. *J Clin Invest* 1987; **79**: 582–587.

90. Kirkpatrick JR, Lawrie JH, Forrest AP, Campbell H. The short pentagastrin test in the investigation of gastric disease. *Gut* 1969; **10**: 760–762.

91. Walsh JH, Richardson CT, Fordtran JS. pH dependence of acid secretion and gastrin release in normal and ulcer subjects. *J Clin Invest* 1975; **55**: 462–468.

92. Moss S, Calam J. *Helicobacter pylori* and peptic ulcers: the present position. *Gut* 1992; **33**: 289–292.

93. Sjovall M, Lindstedt G, Olbe L, Lundell L. Defective inhibition of gastrin release by antral distension in duodenal ulcer patients. *Digestion* 1992; **51**: 1–9.

94. Kihl B, Olbe L. Inhibition of pentagastrin-stimulated gastric

acid secretion by graded intraduodenal administration of oleic acid in man. *Scand J Gastroenterol* 1981; **16**: 121–128.

95. Malagelada JR, Longstreth GF, Deering TB *et al*. Gastric secretion and emptying after ordinary meals in duodenal ulcer. *Gastroenterology* 1977; **73**: 989–994.

96. McHenry L, Jr., Vuyyuru L, Schubert ML. *Helicobacter pylori* and duodenal ulcer disease: the somatostatin link? *Gastroenterology* 1993; **104**: 1573–1575.

97. Levi S, Beardshall K, Haddad G *et al*. *Campylobacter pylori* and duodenal ulcers: the gastrin link. *Lancet* 1989; **i**: 1167–1168.

98. Beardshall K, Moss S, Gill J *et al*. Suppression of *Helicobacter pylori* reduces gastrin releasing peptide stimulated gastrin release in duodenal ulcer patients. *Gut* 1992; **33**: 601–603.

99. Graham DY, Opekun A, Lew GM, Klein PD, Walsh JH. *Helicobacter pylori*-associated exaggerated gastrin release in duodenal ulcer patients. The effect of bombesin infusion and urea ingestion. *Gastroenterology* 1991; **100**: 1571–1575.

100. Moss SF, Legon S, Bishop AE, Polak JM, Calam J. Effect of *Helicobacter pylori* on gastric somatostatin in duodenal ulcer disease. *Lancet* 1992; **340**: 930–932.

101. Kaneko H, Nakada K, Mitsuma T *et al*. *Helicobacter pylori* infection induces a decrease in immunoreactive-somatostatin concentrations of human stomach. *Dig Dis Sci* 1992; **37**: 409–416.

102. Sipponen P, Seppala K. Gastric carcinoma: failed adaptation to *Helicobacter pylori*. *Scand J Gastroenterol Suppl* 1992; **193**: 33–38.

103. Sipponen P. Natural history of gastritis and its relationship to peptic ulcer disease. *Digestion* 1992; **51**(suppl 1): 70–75.

104. Fong TL, Dooley CP, Dehesa M *et al*. *Helicobacter pylori* infection in pernicious anemia: a prospective controlled study. *Gastroenterology* 1991; **100**: 328–332.

105. Moss SF, Calam J. Acid secretion and sensitivity to gastrin in duodenal ulcer patients: effect of eradication of *H. pylori*. *Gut* 1993; **34**: 888–892.

106. Tarnasky PR, Kovacs TO, Sytnik B, Walsh JH. Asymptomatic *H. pylori* infection impairs pH inhibition of gastrin and acid secretion during second hour of peptone meal stimulation. *Dig Dis Sci* 1993; **38**: 1681–1687.

107. El-Omar E, Penman I, Dorrian CA *et al*. Eradicating *Helicobacter pylori* infection lowers gastrin-mediated acid secretion by two-thirds in duodenal ulcer patients. *Gut* 1993; **34**: 1060–1065.

108. Saita H, Murakami M, Dekigai H, Kita T. Effects of ammonia and monochloramine on gastrin release and acid secretion (abstract). *Gastroenterology* 1993; **104**: A183.

109. Golodner EH, Territo MC, Walsh JH, Soll AH. Stimulation of gastrin release from cultured canine G cells by *Helicobacter pylori* and mononuclear cells (abstract). *Gastroenterology* 1992; **102**: A630.

110. Golodner EH, Soll AH, Walsh JH, Calam J. Release of gastrin from cultured canine G-cells by interferon-gamma and tumour necrosis factor-alpha (abstract). *Gastroenterology* 1993; **104**: A89.

111. Figura N, Guglielmetti P, Rossolini A *et al*. Cytotoxin production by *Campylobacter pylori* strains isolated from patients with peptic ulcers and from patients with chronic gastritis only. *J Clin Microbiol* 1989; **27**: 225–226.

112. Crabtree JE, Taylor JD, Wyatt JI *et al*. Mucosal IgA recognition of *Helicobacter pylori* 120 kDa protein, peptic ulceration, and gastric pathology. *Lancet* 1991; **338**: 332–335.

113. Bonnevie O. The incidence of gastric ulcer in Copenhagen county. *Scand J Gastroenterol* 1975; **10**: 231–239.

114. Lambert JR, Lin SK. Prevalence/disease correlates of *H. pylori*. In: Hunt RH, Tytgat GNJ, eds. *Helicobacter pylori: basic mechanisms to clinical cure*. Dordrecht: Kluwer, 1994: 95–112.

115. Graham DY, Lew GM, Klein PD *et al*. Effect of treatment of *Helicobacter pylori* infection on the long-term recurrence of gastric or duodenal ulcer. A randomized, controlled study. *Ann Intern Med* 1992; **116**: 705–708.

116. Karita M, Morshed MG, Ouchi K, Okita K. Bismuth-free triple therapy for eradicating *Helicobacter pylori* and reducing the gastric ulcer recurrence rate. *Am J Gastroenterol* 1994; **89**: 1032–1035.

117. Labenz J, Borsch G. Evidence for the essential role of *Helicobacter pylori* in gastric ulcer disease. *Gut* 1994; **35**: 19–22.

118. Kihira K, Sato K, Yoshida Y *et al*. The effect of the eradication of *H. pylori* on the intractable ulcer. *Nippon Rinsho* 1993; **51**: 3285–3288.

119. Massoomi F, Savage J, Destache CJ. Omeprazole: a comprehensive review. *Pharmacotherapy* 1993; **13**: 46–59.

120. Bodemar G, Walan A, Lundquist G. Food-stimulated acid secretion measured by intragastric titration with bicarbonate in patients with duodenal and gastric ulcer disease and in controls. *Scand J Gastroenterol* 1978; **13**: 911–918.

121. Kikoler DJ, Beck S. Benign gastric ulcers and pernicious anemia. *J Am Osteopath Assoc* 1990; **90**: 535–537.
122. Niemela S, Heikkila J, Lehtola J. Duodenogastric bile reflux in patients with gastric ulcer. *Scand J Gastroenterol* 1984; **19**: 896–898.
123. Gear M, Whitehead R. Chronic gastritis and gastric ulcer. *J Pathol* 1970; **101**: P8.
124. Playford RJ, Hanby, AM, Quinn C, Calam J. Influence of inflammation and atrophy on pancreatic secretory trypsin inhibitor (PSTI) levels within the gastric mucosa. *Gastroenterology* 1994; **106**: 735–741.
125. Wong J, Loewenthal J. Chronic gastric ulcer in the rat produced by wounding at the fundo-antral junction. *Gastroenterology* 1976; **71**: 416–420.
126. Piasecki C. Role of ischaemia in the initiation of peptic ulcer. *Ann R Coll Surg Engl* 1977; **59**: 476–478.
127. Griffin MR, Piper JM, Daugherty JR, Snowden M, Ray WA. Nonsteroidal anti-inflammatory drug use and increased risk for peptic ulcer disease in elderly persons. *Ann Intern Med* 1991; **114**: 257–263.
128. Graham DY, Lidsky MD, Cox AM *et al.* Long-term nonsteroidal antiinflammatory drug use and *Helicobacter pylori* infection. *Gastroenterology* 1991; **100**: 1653–1657.
129. Laine L, Marin Sorensen M, Weinstein WM. Nonsteroidal antiinflammatory drug-associated gastric ulcers do not require *Helicobacter pylori* for their development. *Am J Gastroenterol* 1992; **87**: 1398–1402.
130. Caselli M, Pazzi P, LaCorte R *et al. Campylobacter*-like organisms, nonsteroidal anti-inflammatory drugs and gastric lesions in patients with rheumatoid arthritis. *Digestion* 1989; **44**: 101–104.
131. Jones ST, Clague RB, Eldridge J, Jones DM. Serological evidence of infection with *Helicobacter pylori* may predict gastrointestinal intolerance to non-steroidal anti-inflammatory drug (NSAID) treatment in rheumatoid arthritis. *Br J Rheumatol* 1991; **30**: 16–20.
132. Goggin PM, Collins DA, Jazrawi RP *et al.* Prevalence of *Helicobacter pylori* infection and its effect on symptoms and non-steroidal anti-inflammatory drug induced gastrointestinal damage in patients with rheumatoid arthritis. *Gut* 1993; **34**: 1677–1680.
133. Lanza FL, Evans DG, Graham DY. Effect of *Helicobacter pylori*

infection on the severity of gastroduodenal mucosal injury after the acute administration of naproxen or aspirin to normal volunteers. *Am J Gastroenterol* 1991; **86**: 735–737.

134. Loeb DS, Talley NJ, Ahlquist DA *et al.* Long-term nonsteroidal anti-inflammatory drug use and gastroduodenal injury: the role of *Helicobacter pylori. Gastroenterology* 1992; **102**: 1899–1905.

135. Hudson N, Taha AS, Sturrock RD *et al.* The influence of *Helicobacter pylori* colonisation on gastroduodenal ulceration in patients on non-steroidal anti-inflammatory drugs (abstract). *Gut* 1992; **33**(suppl. 1): S42.

136. Martin DF, Montgomery E, Dobek AS, Patrissi GA, Peura DA. *Campylobacter pylori*, NSAIDs, and smoking: risk factors for peptic ulcer disease. *Am J Gastroenterol* 1989; **84**: 1268–1272.

137. Dixon MF, O'Connor HJ, Axon AT *et al.* Reflux gastritis: distinct histopathological entity? *J Clin Pathol* 1986; **39**: 524–530.

138. Taha AS, Nakshabendi I, Lee FD *et al.* Chemical gastritis and *Helicobacter pylori* related gastritis in patients receiving non-steroidal anti-inflammatory drugs: comparison and correlation with peptic ulceration. *J Clin Pathol* 1992; **45**: 135–139.

139. Bianchi Porro G, Parente F. Non-ulcer dyspepsia and related conditions. In: Calam J, ed. *Baillière's Clinical Gastroenterology: Helicobacter pylori*. London: Baillière Tindall, 1995: **9**: 549–562.

140. Thompson WG, Heaton KW. Functional bowel disorders in apparently healthy people. *Gastroenterology* 1980; **79**: 283–288.

141. Anonymous. Management of dyspepsia: report of a working party. *Lancet* 1988; **i**: 576–579.

142. Lagarde SP, Spiro HM. Non-ulcer dyspepsia. *Clin Gastroenterol* 1984; **13**: 437–446.

143. Talley NJ, Weaver AL, Tesmer DL, Zinsmeister AR. Lack of discriminant value of dyspepsia subgroups in patients referred for upper endoscopy. *Gastroenterology* 1993; **105**: 1378–1386.

144. Klauser AG, Voderholzer WA, Knesewitsch PA *et al.* What is behind dyspepsia? *Dig Dis Sci* 1993; **38**: 147–154.

145. Graham DY, Smith JL, Patterson DJ. Why do apparently healthy people use antacid tablets? *Am J Gastroenterol* 1983; **78**: 257–260.

146. Manning AP, Thompson WG, Heaton KW, Morris AF. Towards positive diagnosis of the irritable bowel. *Br Med J* 1978; **ii**: 653–654.

147. Talley NJ. Spectrum of chronic dyspepsia in the presence of the irritable bowel syndrome. *Scand J Gastroenterol Suppl* 1991; **182**: 7–10.
148. Talley NJ, Zinsmeister AR, Schleck CD, Melton LJ. Dyspepsia and dyspepsia subgroups: a population-based study. *Gastroenterology* 1992; **102**: 1259–1268.
149. Sielaff F. Coincidence between chronic dyspepsia and irritable bowel syndrome (abstract). *Eur J Gastroenterol Hepatol* 1995; **2**(suppl): S105–S106.
150. Rokkas T, Pursey C, Uzoechina E *et al*. *Campylobacter pylori* and non-ulcer dyspepsia. *Am J Gastroenterol* 1987; **82**: 1149–1152.
151. Pettross CW, Appleman MD, Cohen H *et al*. Prevalence of *Campylobacter pylori* and association with antral mucosal histology in subjects with and without upper gastrointestinal symptoms. *Dig Dis Sci* 1988; **33**: 649–653.
152. Morris A, Nicholson G. Ingestion of *Campylobacter pyloridis* causes gastritis and raised fasting gastric pH. *Am J Gastroenterol* 1987; **82**: 192–199.
153. Dooley CP, Cohen H, Fitzgibbons PL *et al*. Prevalence of *Helicobacter pylori* infection and histologic gastritis in asymptomatic persons. *N Engl J Med* 1989; **321**: 1562–1566.
154. Tucci A, Corinaldesi R, Stanghellini V *et al*. *Helicobacter pylori* infection and gastric function in patients with chronic idiopathic dyspepsia. *Gastroenterology* 1992; **103**: 768–774.
155. Loffeld RJ, Potters HV, Stobberingh E *et al*. *Campylobacter* associated gastritis in patients with non-ulcer dyspepsia: a double blind placebo controlled trial with colloidal bismuth subcitrate. *Gut* 1989; **30**: 1206–1212.
156. Goh KL, Parasakthi N, Peh SC *et al*. *Helicobacter pylori* infection and non-ulcer dyspepsia: the effect of treatment with colloidal bismuth subcitrate. *Scand J Gastroenterol* 1991; **26**: 1123–1131.
157. Marshall BJ, Valenzuela JE, McCallum RW *et al*. Bismuth subsalicylate suppression of *Helicobacter pylori* in nonulcer dyspepsia: a double-blind placebo-controlled trial. *Dig Dis Sci* 1993; **38**: 1674–1680.
158. Patchett S, Beattie S, Leen E *et al*. Eradicating *Helicobacter pylori* and symptoms of non-ulcer dyspepsia. *Br Med J* 1991; **303**: 1238–1240.
159. McCarthy C, Patchett S, Collins RM *et al*. Long term prospective study of *Helicobacter pylori* in nonulcer dyspepsia. *Dig Dis Sci* 1995; **40**: 114–119.

160. Kerlin P. Postprandial antral hypomotility in patients with idiopathic nausea and vomiting. *Gut* 1989; **30**: 54–59.

161. Malagelada JR, Stanghellini V. Manometric evaluation of functional upper gut symptoms. *Gastroenterology* 1985; **88**: 1223–1231.

162. Wegener M, Borsch G, Schaffstein J *et al*. Are dyspeptic symptoms in patients with *Campylobacter pylori*-associated type B gastritis linked to delayed gastric emptying? *Am J Gastroenterol* 1988; **83**: 737–740.

163. Pieramico O, Ditschuneit H, Malfertheiner P. Gastrointestinal motility in patients with non-ulcer dyspepsia: a role for *Helicobacter pylori* infection? *Am J Gastroenterol* 1993; **88**: 364–368.

164. Ormand JE, Talley NJ, Shorter RG *et al*. Prevalence of *Helicobacter pylori* in specific forms of gastritis. Further evidence supporting a pathogenic role for *H. pylori* in chronic nonspecific gastritis. *Dig Dis Sci* 1991; **36**: 142–145.

165. Wolfsen HC, Carpenter HA, Talley NJ. Ménétrier's disease: a form of hypertrophic gastropathy or gastritis? *Gastroenterology* 1993; **104**: 1310–1319.

166. Stolte M, Batz C, Eidt S. Giant fold gastritis – a special form of *Helicobacter pylori* associated gastritis. *Z Gastroenterol* 1993; **31**: 289–293.

167. Bayerdorffer E, Ritter MM, Hatz R *et al*. Healing of protein losing hypertrophic gastropathy by eradication of *Helicobacter pylori* – is *Helicobacter pylori* a pathogenic factor in Ménétrier's disease? *Gut* 1994; **35**: 701–704.

168. McCormick PA, Sankey EA, Cardin F *et al*. Congestive gastropathy and *Helicobacter pylori*: an endoscopic and morphometric study. *Gut* 1991; **32**: 351–354.

169. Guslandi M, Sorghi M, Foppa L, Tittobello A. Congestive gastropathy versus chronic gastritis: a comparison of some pathophysiological aspects. *Digestion* 1993; **54**: 160–162.

170. Parkin DM, Pisani P, Ferlay J. Estimates of the worldwide incidence of eighteen major cancers in 1985. *Int J Cancer* 1993; **54**: 594–606.

171. Munoz N. Descriptive epidemiology of gastric cancer. In: Reed RI, Hill MJ, eds. *Gastric carcinogenesis*. Amsterdam: Excerpta Medica, 1993: 51–69.

172. Barker DJ, Coggon D, Osmond C, Wickham C. Poor housing in childhood and high rates of stomach cancer in England and Wales. *Br J Cancer* 1990; **61**: 575–578.

173. Correa P, Fox J, Fontham E *et al. Helicobacter pylori* and gastric carcinoma. Serum antibody prevalence in populations with contrasting cancer risks. *Cancer* 1990; **66**: 2569–2574.

174. Mitchell HM, Li YY, Hu PJ et al. Epidemiology of *Helicobacter pylori* in southern China: identification of early childhood as the critical period for acquisition. *J Infect Dis* 1992; **166**: 149–153.

175. Palli D, Decarli A, Cipriani F *et al. Helicobacter pylori* antibodies in areas of Italy at varying gastric cancer risk. *Cancer Epidemiol Biomarkers Prev* 1993; **2**: 37–40.

176. Sierra R, Munoz N, Pena AS *et al.* Antibodies to *Helicobacter pylori* and pepsinogen levels in children from Costa Rica: comparison of two areas with different risks for stomach cancer. *Cancer Epidemiol Biomarkers Prev* 1992; **1**: 449–454.

177. Anonymous. Epidemiology of, and risk factors for, *Helicobacter pylori* infection among 3194 asymptomatic subjects in 17 populations. The EUROGAST Study Group. *Gut* 1993; **34**: 1672–1676.

178. Forman D, Webb PM. *H. pylori* and gastric cancer: the significance of the problem. In: Hunt RH, Tytgat GNJ, eds. *Helicobacter pylori: basic mechanisms to clinical cure.* Dordrecht: Kluwer Academic, 1994: 461–468.

179. Forman D, Newell DG, Fullerton F *et al.* Association between infection with *Helicobacter pylori* and risk of gastric cancer: evidence from a prospective investigation. *Br Med J* 1991; **302**: 1302–1305.

180. Parsonnet J, Friedman GD, Vandersteen DP *et al. Helicobacter pylori* infection and the risk of gastric carcinoma. *N Engl J Med* 1991; **325**: 1127–1131.

181. Nomura A, Stemmermann GN, Chyou PH et *al. Helicobacter pylori* infection and gastric carcinoma among Japanese Americans in Hawaii. *N Engl J Med* 1991; **325**: 1132–1136.

182. Grigioni WF, D'errico A, Milani M *et al.* Early gastric cancer. Clinico-pathological analysis of 125 cases of early gastric cancer (EGC). *Acta Pathol Jpn* 1984; **34**: 979–989.

183. Correa P, Cuello C, Fajardo LF *et al.* Diet and gastric cancer: nutrition survey in a high-risk area. *J Natl Cancer Inst* 1983; **70**: 673–678.

184. Ihamaki T, Sipponen P, Varis K, Kekki M, Siurala M. Characteristics of gastric mucosa which precede occurrence of gastric malignancy: results of long-term follow-up of three family samples. *Scand J Gastroenterol Suppl* 1991; **186**: 16–23.

185. Parsonnet J, Vandersteen D, Goates J *et al. Helicobacter pylori*

infection in intestinal- and diffuse-type gastric adeno-carcinomas [published erratum appears in *J Natl Cancer Inst* 1991; **83**(12): 881]. *J Natl Cancer Inst* 1991; **83**: 640–643.

186. Mirvish SS. Experimental evidence for inhibition of N-nitroso compound formation as a factor in the negative correlation between vitamin C consumption and the incidence of certain cancers. *Cancer Res* 1994; **54**: 1948s–1951s.

187. Correa P. Is gastric carcinoma an infectious disease? (editorial; comment). *N Engl J Med* 1991; **325**: 1170–1171.

188. Feig DI, Reid TM, Loeb LA. Reactive oxygen species in tumorigenesis. *Cancer Res* 1994; **54**: 1890s–1894s.

189. Isaacson PG. Lymphomas of mucosa-associated lymphoid tissue (MALT). *Histopathology* 1990; **16**: 617–619.

190. Wotherspoon AC, Ortiz Hidalgo C, Falzon MR, Isaacson PG. *Helicobacter pylori*-associated gastritis and primary B-cell gastric lymphoma. *Lancet* 1991; **338**: 1175–1176.

191. Clarke CA, Edwards JW, Haddock DRW, Howel Evans AW, McConnell RB, Sheppard PM. ABO blood groups and secretor character in duodenal ulcer. *Br Med J* 1956; **ii**: 725–731.

192. Muotiala A, Helander IM, Pyhala L, Kosunen TU, Moran AP. Low biological activity of *Helicobacter pylori* lipopoly-saccharide. *Infect Immun* 1992; **60**: 1714–1716.

193. Aird I, Bentall HH, Mehigan JA, Roberts JAF. The blood groups in relation to peptic ulceration and carcinoma of the colon, rectum, breast and bronchus. *Br Med J* 1954; **ii**: 315–321.

194. Blaser MJ, Perez-Perez GI, Kleanthous H *et al.* Infection with *Helicobacter pylori* strains possessing cagA is associated with increased risk of developing adenocarcinoma of the stomach among Japanese-Americans in Hawaii (abstract). *Am J Gastroenterol* 1994; **89**: 1356.

195. Hansson LE, Baron J, Nyren O *et al.* Tobacco, alcohol and the risk of gastric cancer. A population-based case-control study in Sweden. *Int J Cancer* 1994; **57**: 26–31.

4

Diagnosis of infection

INTRODUCTION

Historically, *H. pylori* was first detected by histology, then as gastric urease and finally by culture. Clinical diagnosis was initially based upon developments of these three observations. Each has its advantages. Histology indicates the state of the gastric mucosa, the biopsy urease test is cheap and convenient and culture indicates the bacterium's sensitivity to antibiotics. Outside research centres most clinicians rely on the biopsy urease test, which is quite adequate so long as it is done properly and its limitations are appreciated. Of the non-invasive tests, the urea breath test is most accurate, but it is much less convenient than serology which now provides rapid clinic-room diagnosis. This chapter will describe how to set up and do the different tests, and discuss their relative merits.

Two points apply to all diagnostic methods.

- If you are asking if eradication has been successful, the test should be delayed for at least 4 weeks after the end of therapy [1], and at least 6 months in the case of serology [2].
- The accuracy of each test should be audited against other tests before it is adopted locally.

INVASIVE TESTS

Introduction

Biopsy-based tests are the obvious choice if endoscopy is being done. However, it is important to appreciate two potential sources of false-negative results. Firstly, the uneven distribution of *H. pylori* in the stomach leads to sampling errors. This is especially likely if there is muscosal atrophy with or without intestinal metaplasia [3], because bacterial growth may be less when acid is very scanty and the bacterium cannot colonize intestinal-type mucosa [3]. Sampling errors are diminished by testing multiple biopsies. Secondly, there is the effect of therapy. Antibacterials, including bismuth, can greatly decrease the number of *H. pylori* bacteria, even if they are not going to eradicate the infection [4]. Therefore antibacterials should be discontinued at least 1 month before the endoscopy. Bismuth remains in the body for 3 months after the end of therapy [5]. False-negative results after bismuth therapy may therefore have contributed to the relatively high relapse rates in early eradication studies [6]. Administration of drugs which suppress acid secretion can also interfere with the detection of *H. pylori* in the stomach. Proton pump inhibitors have a direct antibacterial effect on *H. pylori* [7]. They also inhibit its enzyme urease [8], so that the biopsy urease and urea breath tests may give false-negative results. Suppression of acid secretion may decrease the number of *H. pylori* bacteria in the stomach by creating an unfavourably neutral environment. Interestingly, *H. pylori* responds to suppression of acid secretion by moving from the gastric antrum into the proximal stomach [9,10]. Therefore, drugs which suppress acid secretion should be stopped at least 2 weeks before the endoscopy.

H. pylori bacteria are normally most abundant in the gastric antrum, which is quite variable in extent, so it is usual to take biopsies 1–2 cm proximal to the pyloric ring. As a rule of thumb three biopsies should be taken and put into more than one test. Further biopsies should be taken from the gastric fundus if the patient has recently received a proton pump inhibitor.

The biopsy urease test

The biopsy urease test depends on *H. pylori*'s enzyme urease. Several other bacteria produce urease enzymes [11,12]. These include some, such as *Proteus* and *Klebsiella* spp., which can grow in the achlorhydric antrum [13]. However, *H. pylori*'s urease is unusually potent [14] and abundant. The enzyme urease digests urea to produce carbon dioxide and ammonium ions with net production of alkali.

$$NH_2 - CO - NH_2 + H_2O \rightarrow CO_2 + 2NH_3$$

Then, spontaneously at neutral pH,

$$NH_3 + H_2O \rightarrow NH_4^+ + OH^-$$

The production of alkali changes the colour of the pH indicator phenol red from yellow to red, indicating a positive result [15].

In clinical practice the biopsy urease test can be done using the familiar commercial CLOtest® or, more cheaply, with 'in-house' solutions.

The CLO test® (Plate 8)

This test was developed by Barry Marshall [16], working with his father, who is a chemist. Prototypes were made in the Marshall's family kitchen in Perth, with the forbearance of Mrs Marshall. In practice, one or two biopsies are pushed into the gel. It is important to push them right into the gel so that an antibacterial agent present in it will prevent growth of *H. pylori* and other bacteria during incubation. The kit is re-sealed and kept in a warm place at 30–40°C (or endoscopist's pocket) for the next 3 hours, and then at room temperature (20°C) for the rest of a 24 h period.

The result is positive when the gel changes from yellow to pink, but note the following.

- Uninfected biopsies may appear slightly pink when they are first put into the gel, particularly if blood or alkaline bile are present. Ignore this: the result is only positive if the pink area subsequently deepens in colour or expands.
- The CLO test® is read at intervals for 24 h, for example at 20 min and then at 1, 3 and 24 h.
- A positive result may be indicated by an expanding pink zone around the biopsy, or the gel may gradually change to a deep orange followed by a magenta colour. If there are not many bacteria the colour change may gradually affect the whole gel, rather than being localized around the biopsy. If there is an orange colour at 3 h the test will almost certainly change to the magenta colour overnight.
- False-positive results can occur it tests are read after 24 h.

Specificity

The specificity of the CLO test® is around 97% under ideal conditions. However, false positives may occur if the patient's intragastric pH is neutral or nearly so, as a result of gastric atrophy or drug therapy. This is because neutral gastric juice may contain bacteria, such as *Proteus* spp., which also produce urease [11,12]. Such bacteria are unlikely to give a positive result at 3 h because they produce so little urease. If the clinician suspects that the patient has low acid secretion another test for *H. pylori* should be used.

Sensitivity
Sensitivity is about 75% at 20 min, rising to 90% at 3 h and 95% at 24 h. False negatives may be due to antibacterial therapy or sampling problems. The latter may be reduced by putting two biopsies into the single gel.

McNulty's recipe (Plate 9)
McNulty and her colleagues in Gloucester published an exceedingly inexpensive method which we use routinely [17]. The solution is made up as follows:

Urea 40 g is dissolved in 100 ml of water and kept at 4°C. This is self-sterilizing within three days.

Sodium chloride 5 g, potassium dihydrogen phosphate 2 g and phenol red 0.04 g are dissolved in 1 litre of water and adjusted to pH 7.0 by adding drops of hydrochloric acid or sodium hydroxide. This solution is then divided into 47.5 ml aliquots and autoclaved. When required, 2.5 ml of the urea solution is added one of the 47.5 ml aliquots and 300 µl is dispensed into sterile bijoux bottles. The reaction can also be speeded up by incubating the tubes on a warm plate at 37°C rather than at room temperature. It may also be helpful to crush the biopsy slightly with a disposable swab stick when placing it in the solution. The pink colour is often seen on the swab first. Two biopsies are incubated in the solution for 24 h. A change in colour from yellow to red indicates a positive result. In practice this occurs in about 75% of cases within 2 h, even at room temperature. Sensitivity is 90% and specificity is close to 100%.

The Bart's one minute recipe
The St Bartholomew's Hospital group published a method which gives the result in one minute [15]. The following are put into a capped 1.5 ml Eppendorf tube:

- urea 100 g/l, freshly made up in deionized water and brought to pH 6.8 by addition of dilute hydrochloric acid
- 2 drops of 20 g/l phenol red.

A positive result is indicated by a change in colour from yellow to pink within 1 min of adding the biopsy. The change is rapid because the phosphate buffer is omitted. The advantage is speed.

We have found this test really useful in research projects when we needed to know whether the patient was infected or not before the endoscope was withdrawn . The lack of buffer makes pH of the solution unstable during storage. This is overcome by keeping the tubes in a freezer and thawing them out just before use. Again the sensitivity is 90% and the specificity is close to 100%.

Histology

As a diagnostic method histology has two main advantages. Firstly, it gives information on the histological state of the mucosa and may thus allow the diagnosis of rarer conditions of the stomach, such as eosinophilic gastritis, Crohn's disease of the stomach, Ménétrier's disease, dysplasia and early cancer. Secondly, histology provides a permanent record of the patient's condition.

Biopsies are placed in a fixative such as Bouin's solution or formalin. *H. pylori* bacteria can be usually be identified on staining with haematoxylin and eosin, but the sensitivity of detection with this stain is quite operator-dependent. *H. pylori* bacteria can be seen more reliably with special stains [18] such as acridine orange, modified Giemsa [19], cresyl violet or Warthin–Starry stains [20], but the sensitivity may still be less than 85% [21]. False-negatives are likely to be due to antibacterial therapy and sampling errors. The search for bacteria should be particularly diligent if atrophy is present. *H. pylori* bacteria are absent from areas of intestinal metaplasia. Sampling error is less likely if the histologist appreciates this problem and if two biopsies are examined. The specificity of histological diagnosis is almost 100%. *H. heilmanni* (*Gastrospirillum hominis*) infects the human stomach rarely and might be mistaken for *H. pylori* although its morphology is quite different [22] (Plate 10).

H. pylori should be looked for under high magnification in the gastric mucus, surface epithelium and in the crypts. The bacterium is curved or 'S' shaped and 3–4 μm long. Bacteria can adhere to the epithelium but are almost never seen within epithelial cells. It is possible to identify them by immunohistochemistry or even by *in situ* hybridization. The former might be useful when infection is suspected but bacteria are not seen on routine histology [18].

Clinic-room smears
Of course it is useful to be able to diagnose *H. pylori* infection before the patient leaves the endoscopy clinic. One way of achieving this is

to crush, or more usually to rub a biopsy on to a glass slide, and then to look for *H. pylori* bacteria either using a dark-field microscope or an ordinary microscope after staining with methylene blue, acridine orange or Gram stain. The literature indicates that *H. pylori* infection can be accurately diagnosed in this way [23], but the approach has not become popular. This is presumably because most endoscopy units lack a microscope and gastroenterologists are not used to identifying bacteria in this way. A Gram-stained smear may be performed in the microbiology laboratory, in addition to performing cultures of *H. pylori*.

Culture

Culture is probably the most difficult approach to the diagnosis of *H. pylori*. The advantages are that it is highly specific and that the antibiotic sensitivity of the patient's strain can be determined. Of course, this is only important if it affects the choice of eradication regimen. In practice this is not usually the case because eradication is successful in about 90% of patients given standard therapy. Culture generally produces the highest proportion of false-negative results, but sensitivity can be increased by attention to technical details: the forceps must be clean but free from antiseptic. Optimal results are obtained using two biopsies and a transport medium such as Stewart's [24] or Portagerm-pylori® (BioMerieux) [25] kept at 4–10°C until samples are processed [24]. Culture is under micro-aerophilic conditions at 37°C. Media may be non-selective, based on blood or chocolate blood agar, or selective, such as Skirrows's or Glupczynski's Brussels *Campylobacter* medium (Figure 4.1). Sensitivity is increased to over 95% by using one of each [26]. Small transparent colonies appear within 3–4 days, but sometimes later. When *H. pylori* is grown on blood agar containing 40 mg/l of tetrazolium chloride the colonies take on a golden hue which facilitates diagnosis [27].

Identification may be confirmed by testing for the bacterium's enzymes, which include urease, oxidase, catalase and gamma-glutamyl transpeptidase [28]. In the light of current clinical practice it is worth testing for resistance to metronidazole and clarithromycin. Minimum inhibitory concentrations are conveniently determined by placing E-strips®, which contain a range of antibiotic concentrations, on to the culture plate. Amoxycillin is often used in treatment but resistance to it has not so far been encountered.

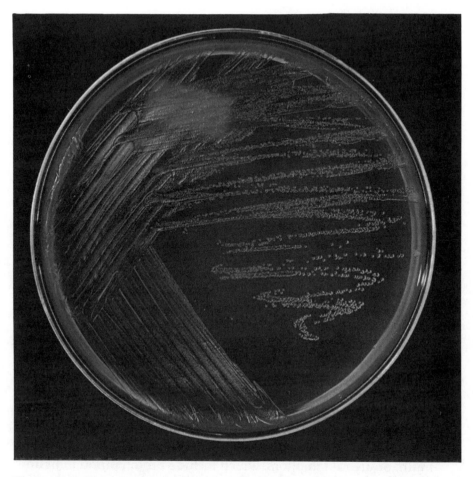

Figure 4.1 The clonal morphology of *H. pylori* grown on a blood-agar-based medium. (Source: provided by Dr R.J. Owen.)

NON-INVASIVE TESTS

The urea breath test (Figure 4.2)

This ingenious test was invented independently by David Graham's group in Houston, TX [29] and in Ipswich, UK by Duncan Bell and colleagues [30]. Atherton and Spiller provide a recent review [31]. The breath test, like the biopsy urease test, is based on *H. pylori*'s unusually potent enzyme urease. The patient drinks urea containing a labelled carbon atom. The appearance of labelled carbon dioxide in the breath indicates that infection is present (Figure 4.3).

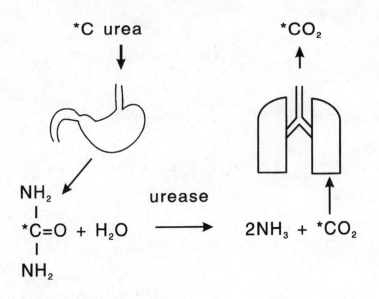

Figure 4.2 The biochemical basis of the urea breath test.

Sensitivity is excellent because the whole stomach is sampled. However users should be aware that false-negative results can occur if the patient has recently been given antibacterials including bismuth, or urease inhibitors, which include proton pump inhibitors and bismuth [9] (Chapter 5). The urease breath test is excellent for determining whether eradication therapy has been successful, so long as it is used at least 1 month after the end of therapy. Indeed it has been adopted as the gold standard for this purpose in clinical trials. Specificity is also high, but there are two potential pitfalls. Firstly, feeble ureases of oral bacteria can produce a small early rise in exhaled CO_2 tracer, but this is over by 20 min. Secondly, the gastric bacteria in patients who secrete little or no acid can produce a weak late rise in exhaled CO_2 tracer [32]. As a non-invasive test for clinical practice the urea breath test is in competition with serology. In this context the urea breath test is more accurate, but less convenient. The patient has to attend fasting and wait to give the breath sample. The result is not available before the patient leaves the clinic unless the unit is unusually well organized or lavishly equipped!

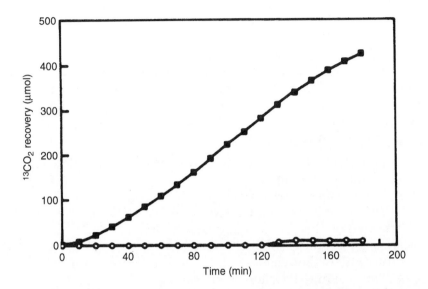

Figure 4.3 Recovery of $^{13}CO_2$ from the breath of an uninfected individual (open circles) and a patient who is infected with *H. pylori* (solid squares) after administration of a test meal containing [^{13}C]urea. (*Source*: from reference 29, with permission.)

If you want to use this method you have a choice between purchasing the carbon-13-based kit from BSIA and following the instructions or setting up a carbon-14-based in-house method, which takes a little organizing but is considerably cheaper. Some simple protocols are given below, after an explanation of the pros and cons.

Aspects of test design
Most urea breath tests have been designed by academics and it is helpful to understand the thought processes that lead to the different protocols.
  1. [^{13}C] or [^{14}C]urea? The rich man's choice is [^{13}C]urea, which is non-radioactive but more expensive and requires commercial off-site analysis of breath. Paupers can use [^{14}C]urea, which is radio-active, but the dose is tiny and [^{14}C]urea is inexpensive and can usually be measured in-house.
  2. The dose? There is a trend to reduce the dose in order to minimize the cost and, in the case of carbon-14, the dose of radiation. The idea is to find the minimum dose that still gives accurate results.

3. Whether to give a meal before the urea? This was done in the first tests in order to delay gastric emptying so as to keep the urea in the stomach for longer. Most people still give a meal, but others seem to get equally accurate results without doing so.

4. When to collect breath samples? Here there is slight conflict between the convenience of taking a single sample early and the possibly increased accuracy of taking multiple samples. In practice most groups have now settled into one of two protocols:

- Protocol 1: with a meal
  - Time 0 min: Meal consumed; baseline breath sample at either
  - − 5 min or + 5 min
  - Time 10 min: Urea ingested
  - Time 40 min: Second breath sample

Variations on this protocol are used by Graham [29,33], Bell [30], Logan [34] and Rauws [35].

- Protocol 2: without a meal
  - Time − 5 min: Baseline breath sample
  - Time 0 min: Urea ingested
  - Time 20 min: Second breath sample

Variations on this protocol are used by Marshall [36,37] and Bardhan [38].

5. To roll or not to roll? It was initially recommended that patients lie first on one side and then on the other for a couple of minutes after taking their dose of urea, in order to distribute the dose around the inside of the stomach. This is reasonable if beds are available but is inconvenient for multiple outpatients. In fact there is no evidence that it helps and both Bell and Graham have stopped doing it. Their patients remain seated throughout.

6. How to calculate the results and what is the upper limit of normal? This differs between the carbon-13- and carbon-14- based tests. In-house methods should be validated locally.

The [^{14}C]urea breath test
[^{14}C]urea is cheaper than [^{13}C]urea and $^{14}CO_2$ can be detected using a beta-counter. If your hospital already has a beta-counter there is strong economic case for setting up the carbon-14 method in-house. The first stated disadvantage of carbon-14 is that it is radioactive. It is a good general principal to avoid irradiation whenever possible, but the dose involved in this test really is tiny [39]. A second disadvantage is that there is no kit for the [^{14}C]urea version. This should not be a big problem but busy clinicians may prefer to pay

extra for a kit rather than spending time setting up an 'in-house' method. Barry Marshall is currently developing a [^{14}C]urea-based kit but it is not yet available. A third feature of the [^{14}C]urea breath test is that it is necessary to collect a fixed amount of CO_2 in order to calculate $^{14}CO_2$/total CO_2. This is not necessary with the carbon-13-based method because the mass spectrometer measures both $^{13}CO_2$ **and** $^{12}CO_2$ to provide the ratio. The physical half-life of carbon-14 is 5000 years so radioactive decay is not a problem!

The doses of [^{14}C]urea used initially by different groups varied between 100 and 185 kBq. Bardhan's group recently described a 'mini-dose' method which uses 37 kBq (1 µCi) (see below), but the dose of irradiation is so low anyway that the 'mini-dose' is optional. For instance Bell's method, which uses 100 mBq, exposes the patient to irradiation in the range from 4 µSv (microsieverts) in a *H. pylori*-negative male to 8 µSv in a *H. pylori*-positive female. Patients living in certain parts of the United Kingdom would receive this dose from background radiation in 1–2 days. The dose is much smaller than those used in routine radiology. Typical irradiation is 40 µSv for a chest X-ray, 1400 µSv for a plain abdominal X-ray, 4630 µSv for a barium meal and 8740 µSv for a barium enema . About 70% of the administered dose of [^{14}C]urea is excreted unchanged in the urine of uninfected persons. The equivalent figure is about 40% in infected persons. Therefore it is the bladder which receives the highest dose of irradiation during the [^{14}C]urea breath test. Despite the low doses it is advisable for the patient to drink plentifully and to void the bladder frequently after the 40 min breath sample has been taken.

The standard equation for calculation of results is:

$$\frac{\% \text{ of dose recovered} \times \text{patient's weight in kg}}{\text{mmol of } CO_2 \text{ collected}}$$

It is usual to publish results in this form, although in clinical practice it may not be necessary to correct for the patient's weight and the administered dose.

Bell's current protocol
This is as follows [30].

- The patient attends after an overnight fast. An unsweetened drink is permitted for breakfast.
- A baseline breath sample is taken: 2 mmol of CO_2.
- 0 min: 50 ml of Calogen is consumed

- This is followed immediately by 100 kBq of [^{14}C]urea in 20 ml water.
- The patient does not roll, but remains sitting throughout.
- 40 min: A further 2 mmol of CO_2 is collected.

In this method the patient exhales through a tube which incorporates a chamber containing anhydrous calcium chloride. This removes water from the exhaled breath. If water remains it may increase the final volume and make counting less accurate. The calcium chloride is omitted by other groups. The breath is bubbled through a scintillation vial containing 2 ml of 1.0 M benzethonium hydroxide (hyamine) in ethanol plus a trace of the trace of phenolphthalein.

The hyamine traps CO_2. When it is saturated the pH rises and the phenolphthalein changes colour from dark blue to colourless; 10 ml of scintillation fluid is then added and carbon-14 activity is measured by liquid scintillation counting.

A standard equal to 1% of the administered dose is also counted and the activity is calculated as above. It is necessary to establish the cut-off value locally. However, Bell regards the result as negative if the result of the standard equation is 0.4% or less.

The Rotherham mini-dose method [38]

- The patient fasts overnight, then provides a baseline breath sample.
- 0 min: He/she drinks 37 kBq of [^{14}C]urea in 25 ml of distilled water through a straw.
- The patient does not roll but remains seated throughout the test.
- 20 min: 2 mmol of exhaled CO_2 is collected.

No desiccating agent is used, but the tube incorporates a liquid trap and a non-return valve to eliminate the possibility of the patient ingesting the hyamine. The amount of hyamine is the same as in Bell's method, but 4 ml of a 0.5 M solution is used, again with a trace of phenolphthalein. The patient exhales thorough this until its colour changes from dark blue to colourless, which takes 1–3 min. Quench correction is applied to give the result in disintegrations per minute. The recovery of CO_2 is calculated by the standard equation, as above.

Their cut off value at 20 min is 0.55%.

This method has a sensitivity of 98% and specificity of 97%, and 100% agreement with the European standard method.

Some other [^{14}C]urea methods

Several other methods for the [^{14}C]urea breath test have been published [37, 40–43]. Rauws's protocol [35] is very similar to Bell's: 110 kBq of [^{14}C]urea is given after a meal and breath is collected 40 min later. The sensitivity is 95% and specificity is 98%. Bardhan's protocol is actually a low-dose version of the protocol developed by Barry Marshall [36,37]. Marshall uses 185 kBq of [^{14}C]urea without a meal and a single breath sample at 20 min. The sensitivity is 100% and the specificity is 97%.

The [^{13}C]urea breath test

Naturally occurring carbon is predominantly carbon-12, but it contains about 11 parts per 1000 of carbon-13. The ^{13}C/^{12}C ratio is expressed as parts per thousand ('per mil') relative to an internationally accepted standard; PDB calcium carbonate. PDB (Pee Dee Belemnite or Belemnitella americana) is a rock from the Pe Dee formation in South Carolina [34]. The ratio in this rock was chosen because it is close to the natural ratio, and it is taken as 0 per mil. This explains why some basal breath samples have less than 0 per mil of $^{13}CO_2$. In the [^{13}C]urea breath test the patient drinks urea containing [^{13}C]urea and the ratio of $^{13}CO_2$:$^{12}CO_2$ is measured in their breath. A rise in the proportion of $^{13}CO_2$ indicates that the patient is infected. This approach does not expose the patient to radioactivity. However, [^{13}C]urea is relatively expensive and mass spectroscopy generally has to be done by a commercial company. The doses of [^{13}C]urea that have been used vary from 75–200 mg.

   Result is expressed as the change in $^{13}CO_2$ per mil in the breath.

The European method, as used in the BSIA kit

This is as follows.

- The patient attends after an overnight fast.
- Time 0 min: He/she then drinks a meal consisting of 50 ml Ensure (Ross Laboratories, Kent) and 50 ml Calogen (Scientific Hospital Supplies).
- 5 min: Baseline breath samples are collected in triplicate – the patient exhales through a drinking tube with its tip in the bottom of a 10 ml exetainer tube until condensation appears. He/she then continues exhaling, slowly removes the exetainer from the straw and screws on the lid.
- 10 min: The patient drinks 100 mg of [13C]urea dissolved in 50 ml of drinking water. He/she then lies on each side for 2 mins before sitting for the rest of the test.

- 40 min: The patient provides further breath samples in triplicate (i.e. 30 min after ingesting [^{13}C]urea).
- Duplicate breath samples are then posted to BSIA for analysis. The third tube from each collection is kept as a backup.
- Infection is indicated by a rise in $^{13}CO_2$ of >5 per mil.

European standard methods

The above method is satisfactory in clinical practice and studies by BSIA showed a sensitivity of 97% and a specificity of 95% in a group of over 5000 patients tested (Mr P. Johnson, personal communication). The 'European standard method' has evolved [35]. The first version was as described above except that breath was collected into 2 l bags at 5, 10, 20, 30, 40 and 60 min, which were then analysed separately. The second version was identical except that, after collecting the 5 min sample into a 2 l bag, subsequent breath samples were collected every 5 min from time 10 to time 40 min inclusive into a single large reservoir bag, then a single 20 ml sample from this was sent for analysis. In these methods each breath was collected by asking the patient inhale fully, then exhale a single breath into the bag. The sensitivity and specificity of both these methods was > 90%.

Graham's [^{13}C]urea method

Graham's group, who invented the [^{13}C]urea breath test [29], evaluated a protocol which closely resembles the BSIA kit in 1000 patients [33]. Patients attend fasting and drink a can of Ensure pudding (Ross Laboratories, Kent) before taking 125 mg of [^{13}C]urea in 125 ml of distilled water at time 0. A rise in $^{13}CO_2$ of >6 per mil is taken to indicate infection. The accuracy varied slightly with the time of breath sampling. Times are from the time that [^{13}C]urea is given. Sensitivity rose progressively from 95% at 20 min to 99% at 50 min. The specificity was 94% at 20 min, but 98–99% at 30–50 min. Therefore the first suitable time for breath collection is 30 min after taking the [^{13}C]urea.

Use of the urea breath test in special groups of patients

- Uraemia: The [^{14}C]urea breath test discriminated between infected and uninfected patients accurately when the breath sample was taken at 20 min, but later sampling gave false positives [32].
- Children: The [^{13}C]urea breath test is preferred because of the lack of radiation [44].

- After gastric surgery: The [^{13}C]urea breath test is reported to give accurate results in patients who have had a partial gastrectomy [45].

Tests based on antibodies

The easiest way to diagnose *H. pylori* infection in a patient who is not being endoscoped is to test for antibodies to it. Several companies have seized this commercial opportunity and produced diagnostic kits. First to appear were 96-well ELISAs designed to be used in a fully equipped laboratory receiving multiple serum samples. Later ELISAs have improved accuracy because they use more sophisticated antibody preparations. The recent development of rapid clinic-room tests is making serological diagnosis much more accessible to doctors. Against this background most clinicians will not consider developing their own immunological tests, but should understand how the commercial kits work and be aware of the factors which can lead to inaccuracy.

Figure 4.4 shows how ELISAs and related tests work.

The various layers are applied one-by one. Time is allowed for each layer to bind, then unbound material is washed off. The *H. pylori* antigen used has developed from crude sonicates, via acid/glycine extracts, to chromatographically purified or recombinant *H. pylori* proteins. *H. pylori* produces a variety of antigens, which vary somewhat from strain to strain. Furthermore, different

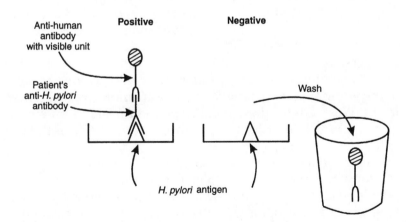

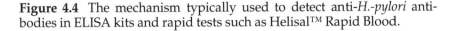

Figure 4.4 The mechanism typically used to detect anti-*H.-pylori* antibodies in ELISA kits and rapid tests such as Helisal™ Rapid Blood.

people produce different amounts of antibody to each antigen. Therefore the best results are generally obtained when a mixture of antigens is used in the test [46]. The tests measure IgG antibodies because *H. pylori* is a chronic infection. If these are present they bind to the antigen on the ELISA plate. Their presence is then detected by adding a 'second antibody' which specifically binds to human IgG. The second antibody is either conjugated to a colour reagent to make it visible or to an enzyme which can produce a coloured product, as in conventional ELISAs. The colour of each well indicates how much antibody is present and is then read on an ELISA plate-reader. The main problem is to decide upon the cut-off between negative and positive results. This generally involves reference to standards which are provided in the kit and used according to the instructions. However in practice it is necessary to validate the method locally against sera from patients whose *H. pylori* status has been established by other methods.

Several factors have been identified that affect the antibody titres.

- First infection: IgG seroconversion occurs 22–33 days after infection [47].
- Antibody titres do not drop significantly until the sixth month after *H. pylori* has been eradicated [2,48].
- Children in the developed world tend to produce lower levels of IgG anti-*H.-pylori* antibodies than adults. Fortunately, Western children have generally had less exposure to other infections so their non-specific antibody binding tends to be low. Therefore when testing children it may be appropriate to reduce the threshold for diagnosis of infection in order to optimize the sensitivity of the test [49,50].
- Conversely, non-specific antibody binding tends to be elevated in certain ethnic groups [51] and in populations living in parts of the world where bacterial infections are more prevalent than in the West. Under these conditions the threshold may need to be increased in order to optimize the specificity of the test [52].
- There appears to be an increased prevalence of false-negative serology in elderly persons [53]. This might be because older people generally produce less antibodies to infections or because they tend have atrophic gastritis, which might decrease exposure of the immune system to *H. pylori*'s antigens. We found that patients with atrophy tend to have lower circulating antibodies to *H. pylori* independent of their age [54].

Sensitivity and specificity of commercial kits
A wide variety of tests are being introduced. These are generally satisfactory but independent testing often shows inaccuracies. It is important to appreciate when choosing a kit that the accuracy figures provided by the manufacturer depend on the population used to validate the assay, as well as how good the particular kit is. There is an awkward group of individuals who have intermediate antibody levels, and accuracy figures can be improved by excluding these prospectively during evaluation of a new assay. Therefore the only satisfactory way to compare kits is by testing the different products on the same population. The results of published comparisons are given in Table 4.1. The differences between the results obtained in different centres underlines the need to validate a method locally, as explained above.

The table illustrates:

- that the same test gives different results in different studies – for example Helico-G gave acceptable results in Holland and the USA, but poor results in Denmark, the UK and Australia;
- that the accuracy of different tests varies quite widely in the same

Table 4.1 Comparative studies; the numbers are sensitivity:specificity

	Jensen [55]	Taha [56]	Hoek [57]	Lamberts [58]	Talley [59]
Country	DK	UK	NL	AUS	USA
Helico-G (Porton Cambridge)	71:74	79:47	82:83	86:65	96:86
GAP-test (Bio-Rad)	77:65	100:30	89:77	83:79	
H. pylori antibodies ELISA (Biometra)	90:74				
Anti-H.-pylori IgG EIA (Roche)	84:74			98:69	
2nd generation H. pylori EIA (Roche)	87:83				
Anti-H.-pylori MTP-assay (Roche)	94:83				
Pylori stat test kit (Whittaker)	90:70				
Pyloriset latex agglutination kit (Orion)	87:65	59:50	68:76	89:69	
Danish in-house ELISA	87:65				
Biolab Malakit		85:50			
HELpTEST (Amrad)				92:77	
Pyloristat (Biowhittaker)					96:94
Premier-H. pylori					88:96

centre – for example the tests from Roche gave the best results in the large study from Denmark.

Why the results vary so much is unclear, but there are several possibilities.

- Kits vary between batches.
- Technique varies between laboratories.
- Bacterial antigenicity varies between local strains.
- The immune response varies between populations.
- The selection of subjects varies between studies.

FUTURE DEVELOPMENTS

Antibodies to specific *H. pylori* antigens

It is relatively easy to develop ELISAs for specific *H. pylori* antigens. For example we may soon be offered measurement of antibodies to the 120–128 kDa product of gene *cagA*. Antibodies to this are present more often in patients with gastric pathology such as ulcers or cancer than in infected persons without these (see Chapters 1 and 3). Unfortunately, not all patients with these conditions give a positive result, so the value of such an ELISA in clinical practice is likely to be limited.

Salivary antibodies

Antibodies to *H. pylori* are present in saliva, but in lower concentrations than in plasma [60]. It is possible to diagnose *H. pylori* infection by measuring salivary antibodies, but there are problems. For example, gingival disease allows circulating antibodies to leak into the saliva, leading to spurious false-positive results.

Clinic-room tests

We already have Helisal rapid blood® (Cortecs, Clwyd), which gives the result from finger-prick blood within 10 min (Plate 11). Smith Kline Diagnostics have developed a test called Flexsure which will soon be available in Europe, but requires serum. These tests are so useful in clinical practice that further developments are inevitable.

Polymerase chain reaction (PCR)

Amplification by PCR makes it possible to detect tiny amounts of *H. pylori's* DNA. PCR is currently under development and may soon be used in diagnosis [61]. Potential benefits include its high sensitivity and the potential to identify toxigenic strains on the basis of the specific genes that they possess (Chapters 1 and 2). When the molecular basis of antibiotic resistance is understood it should also become possible to identify resistant strains by PCR. However there are potential difficulties. PCR detects dead bacteria as well as the living. This, combined with the high sensitivity, increases the danger of cross contamination considerably [61]. Also at present the problem of cross-reaction with other bacteria has not been completely overcome.

PCR could be applied to a variety of samples.

- **Gastric biopsies**: *H. pylori* can be detected by PCR of gastric biopsies [62], but accuracy is still not 100% and there is strong competition from simpler tests such as the biopsy urease test.
- **Gastric juice**: *H. pylori's* DNA can be detected in 96% of samples of gastric juice from infected patients [63]. This might overcome the sampling problems associated with biopsy-based tests, but the patient would still have to be intubated.
- **Saliva**: *H. pylori* can only be detected in the saliva of 40–60% of patients who are infected with *H. pylori* [64,65].
- **Faeces**: Diagnosis of *H. pylori* from stool samples might be the most useful application of this technique, particularly if the strain type can be determined. PCR from stools is technically difficult because faeces contain factors that inhibit the PCR reaction [66]. New clean-up methods may overcome this problem [67]. However, it may be more pleasant to look for antibodies in blood than DNA in faeces!

REFERENCES

1. Weil J, Bell GD, Jones PH *et al.* 'Eradication' of *Campylobacter pylori*: are we being misled? [letter]. *Lancet* 1988; **ii**: 1245.
2. Kosunen TU, Seppala K, Sarna S, Sipponen P. Diagnostic value of decreasing IgG, IgA, and IgM antibody titres after eradication of *Helicobacter pylori. Lancet* 1992; **339**: 893–895.
3. Karnes WE, Jr., Samloff IM, Siurala M *et al.* Positive serum antibody and negative tissue staining for *Helicobacter pylori* in subjects with atrophic body gastritis. *Gastroenterology* 1991; **101**: 167–174.

4. Marshall BJ, Valenzuela JE, McCallum RW *et al*. Bismuth sub-salicylate suppression of *Helicobacter pylori* in nonulcer dyspepsia: a double-blind placebo-controlled trial. *Dig Dis Sci* 1993; **38**: 1674–1680.

5. Gavey CJ, Szeto ML, Nwokolo CU *et al*. Bismuth accumulates in the body during treatment with tripotassium dicitrato bismuthate. *Aliment Pharmacol Ther* 1989; **3**: 21–28.

6. Marshall BJ, Goodwin CS, Warren JR *et al*. Prospective double-blind trial of duodenal ulcer relapse after eradication of *Campylobacter pylori*. *Lancet* 1988; **ii**: 1437–1442.

7. Iwahi T, Satoh H, Nakao M *et al*. Lansoprazole, a novel benzimidazole proton pump inhibitor, and its related compounds have selective activity against *Helicobacter pylori*. *Antimicrob Agents Chemother* 1991; **35**: 490–496.

8. Nagata K, Satoh H, Iwahi T *et al*. Potent inhibitory action of the gastric proton pump inhibitor lansoprazole against urease activity of *Helicobacter pylori*: unique action selective for *H. pylori* cells. *Antimicrob Agents Chemother* 1993; **37**: 769–774.

9. Logan RPH, Walker MM, Misiewicz JJ *et al*. Changes in the intragastric distribution of *Helicobacter pylori* during treatment with omeprazole. *Gut* 1995; **36**: 12–16.

10. Atherton JC, Cockayne A, Balsitis M *et al*. Polymerase chain reaction assay detects the sites at which *Helicobacter pylori* evades treatment with amoxycillin and cimetidine (abstract). *Gut* 1993; **34**(suppl 1): S36.

11. Xia HX, Keane CT, O'Morain CA. Pre-formed urease activity of *Helicobacter pylori* as determined by a viable cell count technique – clinical implications. *J Med Microbiol* 1994; **40**: 435–439.

12. Hu LT, Foxall PA, Russell R, Mobley HL. Purification of recombinant *Helicobacter pylori* urease apoenzyme encoded by ureA and ureB. *Infect Immun* 1992; **60**: 2657–2666.

13. Gray JD, Shiner M. Influence of gastric pH on gastric and jejunal flora. *Gut* 1967; **8**: 74–81.

14. Hu LT, Mobley HL. Expression of catalytically active recombinant *Helicobacter pylori* urease at wild-type levels in *Escherichia coli*. *Infect Immun* 1993; **61**: 2563–2569.

15. Katelaris PH, Lowe DG, Norbu P, Farthing MJ. Field evaluation of a rapid, simple and inexpensive urease test for the detection of *Helicobacter pylori*. *J Gastroenterol Hepatol* 1992; **7**: 569–571.

16. Marshall BJ, Warren JR, Francis GJ *et al*, Blincow ED. Rapid urease test in the management of *Campylobacter pyloridis*-associated gastritis. *Am J Gastroenterol* 1987; **82**: 200–210.

17. McNulty CA, Dent JC, Uff JS, Gear MW, Wilkinson SP. Detection of *Campylobacter pylori* by the biopsy urease test: an assessment in 1445 patients. *Gut* 1989; **30**: 1058–1062.
18. Dixon MF. Histological diagnosis. In: Northfield TC, Mendall M, Goggin PM, eds. *Helicobacter pylori* infection. Dordrecht: Kluwer Academic Publishers, 1994: 110–115.
19. Gray SF, Wyatt JI, Rathbone BJ. Simplified techniques for identifying *Campylobacter pyloridis* (letter). *J Clin Pathol* 1986; **39**: 1279.
20. Warren JR. Unidentified curved bacilli on gastric epithelium in active chronic gastritis (letter). *Lancet* 1983; **i**: 1273.
21. Simor AE, Cooter NB, Low DE. Comparison of four stains and a urease test for rapid detection of *Helicobacter pylori* in gastric biopsies. *Eur J Clin Microbiol Infect Dis* 1990; **9**: 350–352.
22. Dent JC, McNulty CA, Uff JC *et al*. Spiral organisms in the gastric antrum (letter). *Lancet* 1987; **ii**: 96.
23. Zaitoun AM. Use of Romanowsky type (Diff-3) stain for detecting *Helicobacter pylori* in smears and tissue sections. *J Clin Pathol* 1992; **45**: 448–449.
24. Soltesz V, Zeeberg B, Wadstrom T. Optimal survival of *Helicobacter pylori* under various transport conditions. *J Clin Microbiol* 1992; **30**: 1453–1456.
25. Guerreiro S, Pires I, Fernandes E *et al*. *Helicobacter pylori* and bacteriological detection: evaluation of a transport medium 'Portagerm *pylori*' (abstract). *Am J Gastroenterol* 1994; **89**: 1287.
26. Tee W, Fairley S, Smallwood R, Dwyer B. Comparative evaluation of three selective media and a nonselective medium for the culture of *Helicobacter pylori* from gastric biopsies. *J Clin Microbiol* 1991; **29**: 2587–2589.
27. Queiroz DM, Mendes EN, Rocha GA. Indicator medium for isolation of *Campylobacter pylori*. *J Clin Microbiol* 1987; **25**: 2378–2379.
28. Megraud F, Bonnet F, Garnier M, Lamouliatte H. Characterization of '*Campylobacter pyloridis*' by culture, enzymatic profile, and protein content. *J Clin Microbiol* 1985; **22**: 1007–1010.
29. Graham DY, Klein PD, Evans DJ Jr *et al*. *Campylobacter pylori* detected noninvasively by the ^{13}C-urea breath test. *Lancet* 1987; **i**: 1174–1177.
30. Bell GD, Weil J, Harrison G *et al*. ^{14}C-urea breath analysis, a non-invasive test for *Campylobacter pylori* in the stomach (letter). *Lancet* 1987; **i**: 1367–1368.
31. Atherton JC, Spiller RC. The urea breath test for *Helicobacter pylori*. *Gut* 1994; **35**: 723–725.

32. Rowe PA, el Nujumi AM, Williams C *et al*. The diagnosis of *Helicobacter pylori* infection in uremic patients. *Am J Kidney Dis* 1992; **20**: 574–579.
33. Klein PD, Graham DY. Minimum analysis requirements for the detection of *Helicobacter pylori* infection by the ^{13}C-urea breath test. *Am J Gastroenterol* 1993; **88**: 1865–1869.
34. Logan RP, Polson RJ, Misiewicz JJ *et al*. Simplified single sample [13]carbon urea breath test for *Helicobacter pylori*: comparison with histology, culture, and ELISA serology. *Gut* 1991; **32**: 1461–1464.
35. Rauws EA, Royen EA, Langenberg W *et al*. ^{14}C-urea breath test in *C. pylori* gastritis. *Gut* 1989; **30**: 798–803.
36. Marshall BJ, Surveyor I. Carbon-14 urea breath test for the diagnosis of *Campylobacter pylori* associated gastritis. *J Nucl Med* 1988; **29**: 11–16.
37. Marshall BJ, Plankey MW, Hoffman SR *et al*. A 20-minute breath test for *Helicobacter pylori*. *Am J Gastroenterol* 1991; **86**: 438–445.
38. Raju GS, Smith MJ, Morton D, Bardhan KD. Mini-dose (1-microCi) ^{14}C-urea breath test for the detection of *Helicobacter pylori*. *Am J Gastroenterol* 1994; **89**: 1027–1031.
39. Stubbs JB, Marshall BJ. Radiation dose estimates for the carbon-14-labeled urea breath test. *J Nucl Med* 1993; **34**: 821–825.
40. Surveyor I, Goodwin CS, Mullan BP *et al*. The ^{14}C-urea breath-test for the detection of gastric *Campylobacter pylori* infection. *Med J Aust* 1989; **151**: 435–439.
41. Henze E, Malfertheiner P, Clausen M *et al*. Validation of a simplified carbon-14-urea breath test for routine use for detecting *Helicobacter pylori* noninvasively. *J Nucl Med* 1990; **31**: 1940–1944.
42. Debongnie JC, Pauwels S, Raat A *et al*. Quantification of *Helicobacter pylori* infection in gastritis and ulcer disease using a simple and rapid carbon-14-urea breath test. *J Nucl Med* 1991; **32**: 1192–1198.
43. Novis BH, Gabay G, Leichtmann G *et al*. Two point analysis 15-minute ^{14}C-urea breath test for diagnosing *Helicobacter pylori* infection. *Digestion* 1991; **50**: 16–21.
44. Vandenplas Y, Blecker U, Devreker T *et al*. Contribution of the ^{13}C-urea breath test to the detection of *Helicobacter pylori* gastritis in children. *Pediatrics* 1992; **90**: 608–611.
45. Lotterer E, Ludtke FE, Tegeler R *et al*. The ^{13}C-urea breath test – detection of *Helicobacter pylori* infection in patients with partial gastrectomy. *Z Gastroenterol* 1993; **31**: 115–119.
46. Hirschl AM, Rathbone BJ, Wyatt JI, Berger J, Rotter ML.

Comparison of ELISA antigen preparations alone or in combination for serodiagnosing *Helicobacter pylori* infections. *J Clin Pathol* 1990; **43**: 511—513.

47. Morris A, Nicholson G. Ingestion of *Campylobacter pyloridis* causes gastritis and raised fasting gastric pH. *Am J Gastroenterol* 1987; **82**: 192–199.
48. Hirschl AM, Brandstatter G, Dragosics B *et al*. Kinetics of specific IgG antibodies for monitoring the effect of anti-*Helicobacter pylori* chemotherapy. *J Infect Dis* 1993; **168**: 763–766.
49. Crabtree JE, Mahony MJ, Taylor JD *et al*. Immune responses to *Helicobacter pylori* in children with recurrent abdominal pain. *J Clin Pathol* 1991; **44**: 768–771.
50. Czinn SJ, Carr HS, Speck WT. Diagnosis of gastritis caused by *Helicobacter pylori* in children by means of an ELISA. *Rev Infect Dis* 1991; **13**(suppl 8): S700–S703.
51. Webberley MJ, Webberley JM, Newell DG *et al*. Seroepidemiology of *Helicobacter pylori* infection in vegans and meat-eaters. *Epidemiol Infect* 1992; **108**: 457–462.
52. Bodhidatta L, Hoge CW, Churnratanakul S *et al*. Diagnosis of *Helicobacter pylori* infection in a developing country: comparison of two ELISAs and a seroprevalence study. *J Infect Dis* 1993; **168**: 1549–1553.
53. Newell DG, Hawtin PR, Stacey AR *et al*. Estimation of prevalence of *Helicobacter pylori* infection in an asymptomatic elderly population comparing [^{14}C] urea breath test and serology. *J Clin Pathol* 1991; **44**: 385–387.
54. Mathialagan R, Loizou S, Beales ILP *et al*. Who gets false-negative *H. pylori* (HP) ELISA results? (abstract). *Gut* 1994; **35**(suppl 5): S1.
55. Jensen AK, Andersen LP, Wachmann CH. Evaluation of eight commercial kits for *Helicobacter pylori* IgG antibody detection. *APMIS* 1993; **101**: 795–801.
56. Taha AS, Boothman P, Nakshabendi I *et al*. Diagnostic tests for *Helicobacter pylori*: comparison and influence of non-steroidal anti-inflammatory drugs. *J Clin Pathol* 1992; **45**: 709–712.
57. Hoek FJ, Noach LA, Rauws EA, Tytgat GN. Evaluation of the performance of commercial test kits for detection of *Helicobacter pylori* antibodies in serum. *J Clin Microbiol* 1992; **30**: 1525–1528.
58. Schembri MA, Lin SK, Lambert JR. Comparison of commercial diagnostic tests for *Helicobacter pylori* antibodies. *J Clin Microbiol* 1993; **31**: 2621–2624.
59. Talley NJ, Kost L, Haddad A, Zinsmeister AR. Comparison of

commercial serological tests for detection of *Helicobacter pylori* antibodies. *J Clin Microbiol* 1992; **30**: 3146–3150.

60. Clancy RL, Cripps AW, Taylor DC *et al.* The clinical value of a saliva diagnostic assay for antibody to *H. pylori*. In: Hunt RH, Tytgat GNJ, eds. *Helicobacter pylori: basic mechanisms to clinical cure.* Lancaster: Kluwer Academic Publishers, 1994: 342–350.
61. Roosendaal R, Kuipers EJ, van den Brule AJ *et al.* Importance of the fiberoptic endoscope cleaning procedure for detection of *Helicobacter pylori* in gastric biopsy specimens by PCR. *J Clin Microbiol* 1994; **32**: 1123–1126.
62. Van Zwet AA, Thijs JC, Kooistra Smid AM *et al.* Sensitivity of culture compared with that of polymerase chain reaction for detection of *Helicobacter pylori* from antral biopsy samples. *J Clin Microbiol* 1993; **31**: 1918–1920.
63. Westblom TU, Phadnis S, Yang P, Czinn SJ. Diagnosis of *Helicobacter pylori* infection by means of a polymerase chain reaction assay for gastric juice aspirates. *Clin Infect Dis* 1993; **16**: 367–371.
64. Mapstone NP, Lynch DA, Lewis FA *et al.* Identification of *Helicobacter pylori* DNA in the mouths and stomachs of patients with gastritis using PCR. *J Clin Pathol* 1993; **46**: 540–543.
65. Song M. [Detection of *Helicobacter pylori* in human saliva by using nested polymerase chain reaction]. *Chung Hua Liu Hsing Ping Hsueh Tsa Chih* 1993; **14**: 237–240.
66. Mapstone NP, Lynch DA, Lewis FA *et al.* PCR identification of *Helicobacter pylori* in faeces from gastritis patients (letter). *Lancet* 1993; **341**: 447.
67. Saborio G, Castillo G, Luqueno V. Excretion of *Helicobacter pylori* (Hp) in human feces detected by PCR (abstract). *Am J Gastroenterology* 1994; **89**: 1298.

5

Treatment

INTRODUCTION

Eradication of *H. pylori* is a major advance in the management of gastroduodenal diseases. About 95% of peptic ulcers in patients who are not taking NSAIDs are due to *H. pylori* and these ulcers heal faster and are permanently cured by successful eradication therapy (Chapter 3). The same therapy can also heal some lymphomas and may well decrease the risk of gastric cancer if it is given early enough. The development of regimens has progressed at an impressive rate, for example, studies have shown that *H. pylori* can be eradicated from over 90% of individuals by prescribing three capsules and two tablets daily for one week – omeprazole 20 mg, clarithromycin 250 mg b.d. and tinidazole 500 mg b.d. [1] (For further examples see below [1])! However it is currently fashionable to criticize the way in which this achievement has come about. The Americans in particular regard the process with amusement as 'a European cottage industry'. Unfortunately they have been unable to contribute themselves, largely because their lawyers are out of control.

Three points are frequently raised.

1. The trials are much too small
The trials are often criticized because they are too small. This criticism was directed first against studies showing that eradication of *H. pylori* prevented ulcer relapse. Then it was directed against trials comparing different eradication regimens. In fact the size of the trial is unimportant so long as it has been performed properly and then appraised by proper statistical analysis. Smaller studies are only perceived as inadequate because we are used to comparing drugs with very similar efficacy. For example it took a study of 484 patients to show that ranitidine 150 mg is superior to

cimetidine 400 mg in the maintenance of duodenal ulcers (DUs) for 1 year, with a *p* value of < 0.005 [2]. On the other hand, ranitidine 300 mg daily with triple therapy (tetracycline 2 g, metronidazole 750 mg and bismuth subsalicylate containing 755 mg of bismuth, all in divided doses for 2 weeks) could be shown to be superior to ranitidine 300 mg daily alone in the prevention of recurrent ulcers during 1 year, with a *p* value of 0.001 in a study of only 109 patients [3]. A regimen which fails in six out of six patients can be safely identified as useless! On the other hand, now that several 1 week triple regimens have been reported to give about eradication rates of about 90% it is necessary to conduct to large trials to show any differences between them.

2. The major pharmaceutical companies should have been doing big trials
The companies are now undertaking large eradication trials, but have been slow to do so. A cynical view is that they have been afraid to encourage progress that might destroy their ulcer-maintenance markets, but this may not be the whole story or even the main reason. The difficulty is that progress elsewhere has been so fast that by the time a big trial is completed the regimen that was tested has been superseded. Also, it can be difficult for companies to obtain approval for trials of combinations of drugs whose safety profiles were determined when given singly. Trials organized by doctors are not regulated in the same way, so it has been easier for companies to support doctor-driven studies than to organize trials themselves. On the other hand, now that several excellent regimens have been identified we do need the help of the major companies to sort out which are most effective.

3. The results are often only published as abstracts
This is a valid criticism because abstracts are not subjected to the critical peer review that full papers receive. Again the problem arises from the rapid progress. There are plenty of fully published regimens, but these may already be less attractive for clinical use than the latest regimens, which have only appeared in abstracts. There are two genuine problems with results presented as abstracts. Firstly the results of a single trial are often presented at different meetings with progressively more patients entered, so that the sum of the n-numbers in each abstract is bigger than the number of patients actually studied. Secondly without a full methods section it may be unclear that the patient group or the method of drug administration

was sufficiently peculiar as to produce an aberrant result. Some German studies have produced excellent eradication rates, but were performed on patients in hospital, where compliance is likely to be higher than in the community. It is also strongly rumoured that one Australian investigator is in the habit of phoning his subjects nightly to check that they have taken their medication. While this is admirable in clinical practice it is likely to give unusually good results in trials. Studies in older people may give high eradication rates with regimens which depend on a high intragastric pH because older people who are infected with *H. pylori* often have subnormal acid secretion anyway due to gastric atrophy (Chapter 3).

ASPECTS OF TRIALS LIKELY TO AFFECT THE OUTCOME

The end point

It is now generally agreed that the success of a therapy should be presented as the percentage of patients in whom the infection is eradicated. The point here is that it is relatively easy to render the bacterium undetectable by biopsy-based tests or a urea breath test while it remains viable within the patient and ready to regrow after the treatment has been stopped. One aspect is that the treatment's antibacterial effect may simply reduce the number of bacteria to a level that the test cannot detect. However, therapies can give false-negative results in more specific ways. Firstly, bismuth [4] and PPIs [5] specifically inhibit the bacterial enzyme urease, so that tests based on this enzyme might fail to detect the infection. Secondly, *H. pylori* bacteria tend to move to the proximal stomach during suppression of acid secretion so that tests based on biopsies of the antrum become inaccurate [6]. In order to avoid false-negative results it has become accepted that eradication should only be diagnosed if the infection is undetectable 4 weeks after the end of eradication therapy [7]. The period of 4 weeks was arrived at by consensus, but has no sound scientific basis. How long it takes for a particular test to resume its normal sensitivity may depend on which treatment was given. In particular, bismuth remains in the body for up to 3 months after therapy [8] and may therefore result in a late false-negative result. This problem is to be suspected when trials give early 're-infection rates' or ulcer relapse rates of more than about 1% during the first year (in patients not taking NSAIDs). This is almost certainly true of the well known studies by Marshall *et al.*, who used bismuth-based triple therapy [9], and the study by

Hentschel *et al.*, which used ranitidine and two antibiotics [10]. Other studies have shown that rates of infection and re-infection in Westernized countries are actually about 0.3–0.5% in adults [11,12]. Of course, there may be exceptions to this rule in under-privileged groups and in developing countries, where re-infection rates are elevated by poor hygiene and sanitation. There has been no general agreement on which tests should be used to diagnose eradication of *H. pylori*, and the biopsy urease test, bacterial culture, histology and the urea breath tests are all used singly or in various combinations. Of these the [^{14}C] and [^{13}C]urea breath tests are regarded as most accurate, particularly because they sample the whole stomach, and are therefore usually regarded as the 'gold standard' for this purpose [13]. Serology is not useful for determining whether eradication has been successful in trials, or convenient for this purpose in clinical practice, because it takes about 6 months for antibody titres to fall significantly [14,15].

Compliance

Compliance has been identified as a major factor affecting the success of eradication therapy. Therefore patients should be fully informed and highly motivated and regimens should be convenient to take and non-toxic. The 'World Congress' triple therapy (see below) has neither of these virtues. When prescribed in our hospital, patients receive 18 tablets to take each day, and at specific times: bismuth (e.g. tri-potassium di-citrato bismuthate, TDB) 120 mg four times a day, 30 min before meals and at night; metronidazole 2×200 mg three times a day with meals and avoiding alcohol; plus tetracycline 2×250 mg four times a day. In addition, about a third of patients experience side effects on this regimen [16]. It is not surprising, therefore, that Graham's group [17] found that compliance was the major determinant of the success or failure of this regimen (Figure 5.1). By comparison, age, gender, type of disease, duration of therapy and the dose of bismuth had no significant effect. Labenz *et al.* found that compliance was also the main determinant of success with a simpler dual therapy regimen [18].

Antibiotic resistance

Many eradication regimens contain one of the nitroimidazoles – metronidazole or tinidazole. Results obtained with such regimens depend on the sensitivity of the patient's bacterial strain to these

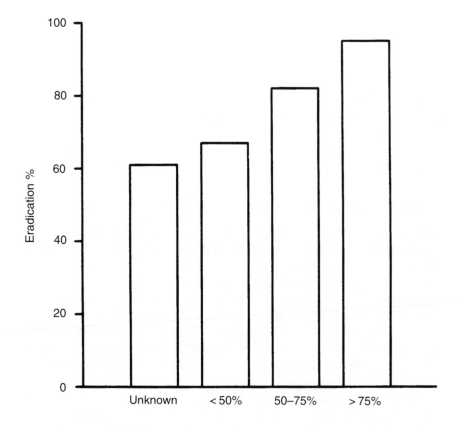

Figure 5.1 The effect of compliance on the rate of eradication of *H. pylori* with triple therapy. (*Source*: drawn from data in reference 17.)

agents, although the importance of this depends on the other components of the regimen (see below). The prevalence of nitroimidazole-resistant strains reflects local usage of these drugs, and varies widely between geographic locations. For instance 74% of strains are resistant to these drugs in central Africa [19], compared with 28% in Europe [20] where such strains are found more commonly in women (35%) than in men (24%) because nitroimidazoles are used to treat *Trichomonas vaginalis*. The prevalence of metronidazole-resistant strains varies widely within the United Kingdom. In our clinic in West London we have a large immigrant community and about 65% of infections are with metronidazole-resistant strains, while in a clinic nearby at the

Central Middlesex Hospital only 34% of strains are resistant to this agent [21]. The proportion of strains of *H. pylori* that were resistant to clarithromycin was 7% in London [22] and 12% in Houston, TX [23]. Fortunately no strains resistant to amoxycillin or tetracycline have been found so far, even in Africa! [19]. For the future it will be important to find regimens that are effective in patients with antibiotic-resistant strains. This is particularly so because failure to eradicate *H. pylori* often leaves patients with a strain that is resistant to nitroimidazoles [24] or clarithromycin [23], if these were used.

Variable responses to drugs

Different patients often absorb, distribute and metabolize drugs at different rates. This can result from disease of major organs such as the liver and kidneys, but is also in some cases genetically determined. Such variability might affect eradication of *H. pylori* but there is little information on this. Of the various drugs used omeprazole has been studied most thoroughly. Savarino examined the dose of omeprazole required to elevate the intragastric pH to 3 or above for 16 hours or more per day [25]. This was achieved in 79% of patients given 20 mg per day and in 94% of patients given 40 mg daily. Differences between the doses required by different patients may be due to variations in the rate of metabolism of omeprazole [26], because the area under the plasma concentration time curve correlates with the degree of acid inhibition [27]. This finding suggests that 40 mg daily omeprazole may be superior to omeprazole 20 mg daily in eradication regimens (see below). Similar considerations probably apply to other components of eradication regimens. For example, the pharmacokinetics of metronidazole been found to vary quite widely between individuals [28] and it would be interesting to know whether this affects the success of eradication therapy.

Disease groups

Graham found no difference between the efficacy of eradication therapy in groups of patients with different diseases when using a bismuth-based eradication regimen [17]. However, as we move to regimens based on suppression of acid secretion, it is likely that the patient's rate of acid secretion will affect the likelihood of eradication. Acid secretion rates tend to be highest in duodenal ulcer disease, intermediate in non-ulcer dyspepsia and lowest in patients with extensive atrophy, such as the elderly, or patients with gastric ulcers. There is already some evidence that this is the case. Labenz *et al.* found higher eradication rates in the elderly, and in patients with severe gastritis or gastric ulcers [18].

Children versus adults

Paediatricians generally use dual therapy consisting of bismuth plus amoxycillin, which gives better eradication rates in children than in adults [29]. The reason for this is unknown, but might be due to a different immune response or less acid secretion after first infection: De Giacomo *et al.* obtained an eradication rate of 68% using tri-potassium di-citrato bismuthate (TDB) (480 mg/1.73 m^2/d) for 1 month plus amoxycillin for the first 2 weeks of therapy [29]. Mahony, Wyatt and Littlewood [30] obtained an eradication rate of 75% using TDB (120 mg b.d. < 10 years; 240 mg b.d. > 10 years of age) for 2 months, plus ampicillin (250 mg q.d.s. < 10 years; 500 mg q.d.s. > 10 years of age) for the first 2 weeks. Israel and Hassall [31] obtained an eradication rate of 100% using bismuth subsalicylate (262 mg q.d.s. < 10 years old; 524 mg q.d.s. > 10 years old) with amoxycillin (250 mg t.d.s. < 10 years; 100 mg t.d.s. > 10 years of age), both given for 6 weeks. Children who had previously failed to eradicate due to the use of monotherapy or poor compliance were given the above dual regimen plus metronidazole (15–20 mg/kg/d in two divided doses) for 4 weeks, but the paper [31] does not state whether this was for the first or the last 4 weeks. However, it is preferable to give children CBS rather than bismuth subsalicylate because it avoids giving a significant dose of salicylate, which is associated with Reye's syndrome in young children.

Sanctuary sites

One explanation for failure of eradication therapy is that *H. pylori* persists in 'sanctuary sites'. For instance, the bacterium was shown by polymerase chain reaction to be evading eradication in over half of the patients, by remaining in the proximal stomach during treatment with cimetidine and amoxycillin [32]. This may be because oral administration of amoxycillin produces higher mucosal concentrations of antibiotic in the antrum than in the gastric fundus [33]. Other sites where *H. pylori* might evade eradication are the periodontal spaces [34], Meckel's diverticulum [35] and the colon [36]. Most of the drugs used to eradicate *H. pylori* are highly effective at a neutral pH, so they will probably kill bacteria in these sites, so long as delivery of the drug is good and the strain is not resistant to the antibacterial agent.

The timing of medication

The times at which medication is taken can affect the success of eradication therapy but this has not been studied in detail. Drug absorption can be affected by meals, but certain aspects are peculiar to regimens for eradication of *H. pylori*. The concentration of drug in the gastric lumen will be diluted if a meal is also present, but the meal might prolong exposure of the bacteria to the drug by delaying gastric emptying. Perhaps more importantly, the buffering effect of food might increase the effect of antibiotics such as amoxycillin by elevating the intragastric pH. Atherton *et al.* showed that amoxycillin suspension given with once-daily omeprazole in dual therapy gave a higher eradication rate when given before, rather than after, meals [37]. Therefore failure of eradication therapy might occur in patients who unwittingly take their medication at the wrong time. Ideally eradication regimens should be robust in this respect, and Atherton *et al.* have now shown that when amoxycillin is given as capsules the timing of antibiotic administration in relation to meals does not affect the *H. pylori* eradication rate [38].

Formulation

Similarly, the formulation of drugs might be particularly important in determining their distribution within the stomach. Weil *et al.* [39] obtained an eradication rate of 54% using TDB liquid with pivampicillin, compared with 0% using the same dose of TDB as tablets with the same dose of antibiotic. This merits further examination because it is currently usual to use bismuth tablets rather than the liquid.

PRINCIPAL AGENTS USED IN ERADICATION

Harris and Misiewicz have recently written a comprehensive review of the efficacy of individual agents and combination therapies in the eradication of *H. pylori* [40].

Bismuth

The heavy metal bismuth is an ancient antibacterial agent that was widely used in the pre-antibiotic era, for instance in the treatment of syphilis. Bismuth is available in several preparations, which seem to have similar properties [41]. The preparation most widely used in Europe is tri-potassium di-citrato bismuthate (TDB). This is available as liquid or tablets. The former was superior in the eradication of *H. pylori* in one study (see above) [39], but is not generally used because it tastes strongly of ammonia and is less convenient than the tablet. TDB is not available in America, where bismuth subsalicylate is used and appears to be similarly effective [42].

How bismuth kills *H. pylori* bacteria is not clearly defined. It is likely to be something of a 'blunt instrument' which acts in several ways. TDB blocks adhesion of *H. pylori* bacteria to epithelial cells, accumulates along bacterial membranes and inhibits the *H. pylori*'s enzyme urease [4]. In addition it acts on the host to stimulates mucosal prostaglandin synthesis and bicarbonate secretion. It also forms a complex with glycoproteins which might protect the epithelium and particularly any ulcerated areas [43].

When it is used alone to heal duodenal and gastric ulcers TDB is, remarkably, about as effective as a histamine H_2-receptor antagonist [44]. It was noted before the discovery of *H. pylori* that bismuth decreases pepsin secretion [45], but without changes in acid output or direct inhibition of pepsin [46]. Furthermore, bismuth improved the ultrastructural appearances of duodenal microvilli while cimetidine did not [47]. It is now interesting to speculate that suppression of *H. pylori* was involved in some of these effects.

In 1981 Martin *et al.* found that remissions of DU disease are considerably longer after they had been healed with bismuth rather than cimetidine [48] (Figure 5.2). No explanation was initially apparent. However this observation has now been confirmed [49] and it seems likely that suppression of *H. pylori* by bismuth contributed to this effect. The far lower relapse rate that Martin *et al.* saw after bismuth seems out of keeping with the eradication rates of about 19% that TDB is now thought to achieve [50]. This might be because Martin *et al.* used liquid TDB, which appears to produce higher eradication rates than TDB tablets [39]. In addition, it is possible that retention of bismuth in the patient's tissues prolongs suppression of the infection [8].

When TDB is taken orally only about 0.2% is absorbed [42], which is fortunate because high circulating levels are neurotoxic. Absorption of bismuth from bismuth subsalicylate is even less [51]. Excretion is via the kidney. Bismuth particles penetrate the antral mucosa [52], and bismuth does accumulate in the body after oral administration so that it is still detectable in the urine 3 months after a 6-week course [8]. The formulation of bismuth affects absorption. For instance, plasma levels are about 100 times higher after TDB than after bismuth carbonate [53]. In practice a short course of TDB appears to be well tolerated. The main side effects are blackening of the stools and occasional nausea. The tongue may be blackened by the liquid but not by swallowing the tablet. Neurotoxicity has only been described in patients who took excessive doses or had impaired renal function, or both [54,55]. Such cases developed an encephalopathy which was reversible on stopping the drug [55].

Proton pump inhibitors

The discovery that proton pump inhibitors (PPIs) can be used in the eradication of *H. pylori* has done much to stimulate the development of new, more convenient eradication regimens. These agents are substituted benzimidazoles and act by selectively inhibiting the hydrogen/potassium ATPase (H^+/K^+ ATPase), which is present in

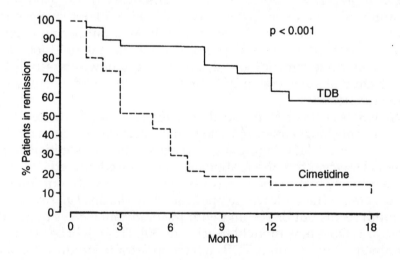

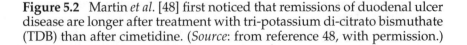

Figure 5.2 Martin *et al.* [48] first noticed that remissions of duodenal ulcer disease are longer after treatment with tri-potassium di-citrato bismuthate (TDB) than after cimetidine. (*Source*: from reference 48, with permission.)

the microtubules of parietal cells and is responsible for pumping protons (H^+ = acid) into the gastric lumen. Because PPIs act in this way their effect lasts for more than 24 hours, while new pumps are synthesized, despite the drug having a short plasma half-life. PPIs are selectively taken up into the acidic environment of parietal cells, where they are converted to a sulphenamide, which inactivates the proton pump by forming disulphide bridges with it [56]. The PPIs currently available in the UK are omeprazole and lansoprazole. These agents offer significantly greater inhibition of acid secretion than histamine H_2-receptor antagonists [57], and are superior to H_2-antagonists in healing of duodenal and gastric ulcers as well as reflux oesophagitis [56].

PPIs have a direct antibacterial effect *in vitro*. However this does not seem to be important in eradication therapy. The role of PPIs in eradication regimens is to suppress the host's acid secretion. This is clear because histamine H_2-receptor antagonists which have no direct antibacterial effect *in vitro* are also effective in eradicating *H. pylori* when given with antibiotics [10]. Antibiotics are far more effective against *H. pylori* when the pH is near to neutral [58,59] and suppression of acid secretion acts by creating these conditions. A lack of acid secretion also discourages the growth of *H. pylori*, perhaps because the bacterium requires some acid to neutralize the alkali that it generates [60]. The direct bacteriostatic effect of PPIs on *H. pylori* can be detected *in vitro* by measuring the minimum concentration of drug which inhibits bacterial growth by 90%; the MIC_{90}. The MIC_{90} of lansoprazole (6 µg/ml) is fourfold lower than the MIC_{90} of omeprazole (25 µg/ml) [61]. The mechanism of this effect is unclear but there may be covalent binding of activated drugs to -SH (thiol) groups on the bacterium's surface. *H. pylori*'s cell membrane contains an ATPase which is inhibited by PPIs in an acid environment [62]. It appears to be of the P-type, which means that it resembles the 'proton pump' of parietal cells rather than the ATPases normally found in bacteria [62]. This ATPase might enable *H. pylori* to maintain the huge proton (H^+) gradients that are present across its cell membrane when it is exposed to gastric acid. Such a role might explain why omeprazole has greater bactericidal activity at pH 5 than at pH 7; the bactericidal activities of omeprazole and lansoprazole were similar at the acid pH [63].

Despite their antibacterial effect PPIs have not been shown to eradicate *H. pylori* from patients unless given with antibiotics. However PPI monotherapy does have quite marked effects on *H. pylori* bacteria within the stomach, which are important because they can cause false-negative test results. These agents decrease the antral density of *H. pylori*, while the number of bacteria in the gastric fundus is unaffected or even increased [6]. Therefore it is advisable to discontinue PPI therapy at least (say) 2 weeks before endoscopy. If PPIs are taken during the few days before endoscopy extra biopsies should be taken from the gastric fundus. Testing should not rely on the enzyme urease because this is inhibited by PPIs [5].

The toxicity of PPIs is low and studies have shown that it is close to placebo levels and similar to rantidine [64]. Patients occasionally experience diarrhoea or a headache. Omeprazole is fully licensed for long-term use although this should now be unnecessary in conditions due to *H. pylori*!

Nitroimidazoles

The nitroimidazoles, metronidazole and tinidazole, act by binding to bacterial DNA. They have proved to be exceedingly valuable in *H. pylori* eradication and are used in most of the regimens which give good eradication rates. Two factors may explain why they are more effective than the many other agents that kill *H. pylori in vitro*. Firstly, their distribution in the body is excellent. They are rapidly distributed to all tissues, and concentrations in saliva are the same as those in the blood [65]. They also appear to pass freely into gastric juice, because metronidazole given intravenously appeared rapidly in gastric aspirates [66]. High concentrations of the drug in gastric juice probably contribute to eradication of *H. pylori*. Drug secreted in saliva and then swallowed may contribute to intragastric concentrations of nitroimidazole. A second advantage of these agents is that, unlike other antibacterials, their effect on *H. pylori* is undiminished at a lower pH [58,59].

Goodwin noticed that nitroimidazole-resistant strains of *H. pylori* appear if a nitroimidazole is given but eradication does not occur [67]. Such strains presumably emerge because of selective pressure during therapy, but it is not clear whether they arise by new mutations during therapy or whether they were present in small numbers at the outset. Nitroimidazoles are widely used to treat anaerobic bacteria and protozoa such as *Trichomonas* and *Giardia*. This gives rise to the pattern of nitroimidizole resistance described above – about three-quarters of strains are resistant in some developing countries in, for instance, Africa [19]. Elevated rates of resistance are found in immigrants from such regions. About 30% of strains are resistant to nitroimidazoles in the West, where women are more likely to have resistant strains than men because of the treatment for *Trichomonas vaginalis* [20]. The biochemical basis for nitroimidazole resistance is being examined. Sensitive organisms reduce nitroimidazoles to a reactive form which causes death through DNA damage [68]. Therefore resistance might be due to less reduction or 'futile' reoxidation of the drug. We found that metronidazole resistance was associated with slower uptake of the drug into *H. pylori* bacteria [68]. Nitroimidazole resistance is not an all-or-none phenomenon so 'resistant' strains may still respond to high doses of these agents. Cross-resistance has been shown between metronidazole and tinidazole which differ only slightly in their structure and kinetic properties [98]. Metronidazole is usually given three times a day while tinidazole is taken once or twice daily. The rapid development of nitroimidazole resistance probably explains why eradication rates are very low on nitroimidazole monotherapy. Of 29 patients treated with cimetidine and metronidazole, one achieved eradication of *H. pylori*, giving an eradication rate of 4% [67]! Furthermore, nitroimidazoles are relatively toxic and poorly tolerated. The unpleasant taste of the tablet itself is avoided by sugar-coating of some preparations such as Flagyl, but this does not eliminate the taste because the drug is secreted in saliva. Other common side effects include nausea, diarrhoea, rashes, headache and drowsiness. Neurotoxicity and leucopenia may occur, but are unlikely to result from the short courses used in *H. pylori* eradication regimens. Some patients suffer a disulfiram-like effect, so alcohol should be avoided. Nitroimidazoles are potentially teratogenic and should be avoided in women who could be pregnant. The side effects of nitroimidazoles provide a good reason for short eradication regimens and fortunately it is now only necessary to take them for one week.

Amoxycillin

Amoxycillin is very widely used in the treatment of *H. pylori*. It is acid-stable and absorbed from the stomach as well as the intestine. Amoxycillin, in common with other penicillins, kills bacteria by preventing the assembly of their cell wall. All isolates are highly sensitive to amoxycillin but eradication rates with amoxycillin monotherapy are only about 23% [69,70]. This is probably because the amoxycillin is much less effective against *H. pylori* when the pH is low [58,59]. Eradication occurs much more frequently if amoxycillin is given with omeprazole [71].

There are conflicting reports on the penetration of orally

administered amoxycillin into the gastric mucosa. McNulty *et al.* [72] achieved bactericidal levels in all of their subjects after giving 500 mg of amoxycillin orally, but Cooreman, Krausgrill and Hengels [33] failed to obtain bactericidal levels in the mucosa of most of their subjects after giving 1 g orally. Levels were particularly low in gastric corpus mucosa [33]. If this is correct it might may explain why *H. pylori* persists in the proximal stomach during treatment with amoxycillin and cimetidine [32]. The side effects of amoxycillin include allergy, monilia and diarrhoea. Pseudomembranous colitis may occur, but is unusual.

Tetracycline

Tetracycline acts by inhibiting bacterial protein synthesis. Few of the latest eradication regimens include this antibiotic, even though a meta-analysis suggested that it is considerably better than amoxycillin when given with bismuth and metronidazole [70]. This is a little surprising because absorption of at least one tetracycline is decreased by chelation with bismuth [73]. Perhaps tetracycline is chelated and then carried into the mucosa with the bismuth particles to provide depot dual therapy? Tetracycline is actively transported into bacteria. Once inside it inhibits protein synthesis by binding to the bacteria's ribosomes. One of the tetracyclines, doxycycline, has been tested and found to be ineffective when given as monotherapy for *H. pylori* infection [74]. Side effects of tetracyclines include gastrointestinal disturbances, erythema and headache. Pancreatitis and pseudomembranous colitis also occur rarely.

Clarithromycin

Macrolide antibiotics exert a bacteriostatic effect by preventing bacterial ribosomes from producing proteins. Macrolides such as erythromycin are effective against *H. pylori in vitro* [59], and erythromycin is secreted in gastric juice [66], but clarithromycin is the only macrolide which has been found to be useful in patients. This may be because it is more potent than the other macrolides. At pH 5.5 it retains anti-*H. pylori* activity [75] (Table 5.1). Tissue penetration is also excellent [76]. Clarithromycin is metabolized extensively on first pass to 14-hydroxyclarithromycin, but this retains activity against *H. pylori*. An interesting finding is that co-administration of clarithromycin with omeprazole increases plasma concentrations of clarithromycin and 14-hydroxyclarithromycin

Table 5.1 The effect of pH on the activity of antimicrobial agents against *H. pylori* (*Source*: From references 59 and *113, with permission)

	MIC_{90} (mg/l)	
	pH 5.5	*pH 7.5*
Ampicillin	0.5	0.06
Penicillin	0.5	0.03
Tetracycline	0.5	0.12
Metronidazole	2	2
Ciprofloxacin	2	0.12
Erythromycin	8	0.06
	pH 5.75	pH 7
Clarithromycin*	0.5	0.03

[77]. Clarithromycin is also the most effective monotherapy for *H. pylori* infection. Graham *et al.* obtained an eradication rate of 42% in 12 patients treated with clarithromycin 250 mg four times daily for 2 weeks [78]. Initial studies of clarithromycin in combination therapies used high doses such as 500 mg thrice daily for 2 weeks [22]. Fortunately it has now been found that 250 mg twice daily for 1 week produces good results in triple therapy (see below). About 10% of clinical isolates tested were resistant to clarithromycin [22,23]. As with the nitroimidazoles there is a tendency for failed eradication to produce clarithromycin-resistant strains [23]. Clarithromycin produces significant side effects including gastrointestinal disturbances, headache, rash, and occasionally elevated liver enzymes. Pseudomembranous colitis can occur [79]. The drug is secreted in saliva and this produces a metallic taste.

COMBINATION THERAPIES

The results of using the various agents alone are described above. The only agent that produces an appreciable eradication rate by itself is clarithromycin and the results obtained [23] with this expensive agent are too low to be useful in clinical practice. Fortunately, better results can be obtained using a combination of agents. How the different agents work together in combination therapies remains open to speculation, but there are several possibilities. Firstly, one drug might create conditions that allow the other to work. For instance, acid-suppressing drugs elevate the intragastric pH into a range where antibiotics become effective. Secondly, one agent might increase the bioavailability of another, as appears to be the case in combinations of omeprazole and clarithromycin (see above). Finally, multiple agents might provide an additive or even synergistic effect on the bacterium itself. In particular one drug may prevent the growth of strains which are resistant to the other, or kill bacteria remaining in 'sanctuary sites' which are inaccessible to the other agent (see above).

Dual therapy regimens

A large number of dual therapies have been assessed, but only two of these have been used extensively in clinical practice. Bismuth plus metronidazole was used in the early days, before better regimens appeared. More recently omeprazole plus amoxycillin received considerable attention and became the first eradication regimen to be licensed in the United Kingdom.

Bismuth plus an antibacterial agent
Bismuth plus an imidazole
Co-administration of bismuth and metronidazole in different regimens is reported to give eradication rates of 38–86%. However, there were few patients in each trial and, more importantly, many studies only included patients with metronidazole-sensitive strains. This was the case in the studies by Bell *et al.* [80], who obtained the highest eradication rate of 80% using TDB 240 mg b.d. and metronidazole 400 mg t.d.s., both taken for 2 weeks. If bismuth was continued for a further 2 weeks the eradication rate rose to 86%. Re-infection rates were higher than expected in these early studies and Bell has pointed out that eradication rates were probably overestimated. This may have been because retained bismuth made the infection undetectable on re-testing (see above). Bismuth plus tinidazole produced eradication rates of 46% [81] and 74% [67]. Historically, interest in this combination waned when it became clear at the 1990 World Congress of Gastroenterology in Sydney that consistently superior results could be obtained by adding amoxycillin or tetracycline (see below).

Bismuth plus a penicillin
Overall, the results obtained using bismuth with penicillins in dual therapy have been poor. A bismuth–amoxycillin combination gave an eradication rate of only 33% [82], but this combination seems to

be more successful in children (see above). Pivampicillin gave an eradication rate of 54% when given with CBS liquid but an eradication rate of 0% when given with TDB tablets [39].

Bismuth with a 4-quinolone antibiotic

This group of antibacterials includes ciprofloxacin, oxacillin and nalidixic acid. An eradication rate of 87% was obtained using CBS 120 mg q.d.s. for 28 days with oxacillin 500 mg q.d.s. for 10 days [83], but the eradication rate was only 40% when the same dose of TDB was used with oxacillin 300 mg b.d. [84].

Bismuth plus furazolidone

Eradication rates of 70% [85] and 100% [86] have been reported with this combination in small studies. However the better figure was obtained in a study in which follow-up consisted of a single antral biopsy! Furazolidone is quite toxic and is not available in the UK.

Comment

Eradication rates of around 70% may be obtained by combining bismuth with nitroimidazoles, furazolidone or oxacillin. The formulation of bismuth merits attention. Bismuth liquid appears to be more effective than bismuth tablets, probably because the liquid is distributed better around the stomach. Penicillins appear to give poor results if acid secretion is not suppressed.

Omeprazole with one antibiotic

Omeprazole and amoxycillin

This combination has received much attention because it is convenient and gives a low incidence of side effects. It was the first regimen to be licensed for eradication of *H. pylori* in the UK. Unfortunately, the main feature of the data on this agent is a perplexing variation between the results obtained in different centres. Some excellent results have been obtained in Germany but elsewhere the results are not as good. This may be related to compliance, which Labenz found to be the most important determinant of success [18]. The results might also be expected to depend upon the patients' rates of acid secretion, which might in turn vary with geographical differences in the prevalence of gastric atrophy.

Eradication rates following administration of omeprazole with amoxycillin for at least 2 weeks vary from 28%, achieved by Logan, Rubio and Gummell [87] in 18 patients given omeprazole 40 mg o.d. and amoxycillin 500 mg q.d.s. for 2 weeks, to Labenz *et al.* [88], who eradicated *H. pylori* from 92% of 13 patients using omeprazole 40 mg b.d. and amoxycillin 1000 mg b.d. for 2 weeks! Somewhere near the middle of this wide range, Unge *et al.* [71] achieved 54% eradication in a double-blind placebo controlled study of 157 patients in which the eradication group received omeprazole 40 mg o.d. for 4 weeks with amoxycillin 750 mg b.d. for the last 2 weeks. The eradication rate was 74% if patients who took less than 90% of their medication were excluded. Therefore the key question is, how can Logan become Labenz without moving to Germany?

Several factors seem to correlate with success *versus* failure, although their roles have not usually been formally tested. Better results have been obtained when omeprazole was given twice, rather than once daily, but this point has not been tested in a randomized trial. Results can be improved by giving more omeprazole. Mannes *et al.* reported a progressive rise from 37% eradication on 20 mg to 85% when 120 mg of omeprazole was taken daily [89]. All the patients took 1 g b.d. of amoxycillin. However, Labenz *et al.* found that increasing the dose of omeprazole from 40 mg to 80 mg daily had no significant effect on the eradication rate [18]. One would expect the effect of the antibiotic to be dose-dependent, and better results are generally obtained when at least 2 g of amoxycillin are given daily. It has been suggested that results might be worse if the patient is on omeprazole before starting the amoxycillin, as in Unge's trial. This was found to be so by Labenz *et al.* [18], although not by another group [90]. Atherton obtained better results when the amoxycillin suspension was given before, rather than after meals [37]. However the difference disappeared when amoxycillin capsules were used [38].

Omeprazole with clarithromycin

Clarithromycin is the most effective single agent in monotherapy (see above) and should therefore be a good companion for omeprazole in dual therapy. Katelaris *et al.* [91] compared omeprazole 40 mg for 2 weeks with either amoxycillin or clarithromycin, both 500 mg t.d.s., and obtained similar eradication rates of 69% and 72% respectively with each regimen. Clarithromycin is much more expensive and moderately more toxic than amoxycillin, and clarithromycin-resistant strains of *H. pylori* have been reported. The Parkside Helicobacter Group have compared different doses of omeprazole with clarithromycin in a high dose of 500 mg t.d.s. In 2-week regimens omeprazole 20 mg gave an eradication rate of 46% [92]. Omeprazole 20 mg b.d. gave a rate of 55% [92], and omeprazole

40 mg daily gave rates of 63% and 80% [93,94]. Other groups have obtained broadly similar results, with eradication rates depending on the dose of both agents and the duration of therapy. The incidence of side effects was relatively high, at 28–66% [22,94]. The commonest complaint is taste disturbance due to excretion of the drug and its metabolite in saliva.

Omeprazole with other macrolides
Eradication rates of 36–52% have been obtained when omeprazole has been used with other macrolides, such as erythromycin [95], azithromycin [96] and roxithromycin [97].

Comment
Dual therapies based on omeprazole and one antibiotic may be simpler to take than triple therapies. They are also less toxic if the antibiotic is amoxycillin. Omeprazole and amoxycillin is one of the few regimens with no apparent risk of producing antibiotic-resistant strains, since resistance of *H. pylori* to amoxycillin has not been reported [98]. However there is alarming variability between the results of different studies using similar regimens. One interpretation is that, in the absence of a drug like metronidazole which works at a low pH, the results depend heavily on whether omeprazole produces a high intragastric pH. This varies from person to person and depends on compliance. At the time of writing attention is turning to one week triple regimens which consistently produce high eradication rates.

Triple therapies

The most effective way to eradicate *H. pylori* is still with triple therapy because eradication rates are higher and consistently so in trials. However there is still a lack of randomized trials which directly compare triple and dual regimens on an intention-to-treat basis. These are needed because the complexity of triple regimens might seriously decrease compliance in 'the real world'. In this context the new short simple triple therapies based on omeprazole and two antibiotics are most welcome (see below).

'World congress triple therapy'
A working party at the 1990 World Congress of Gastroenterology in Sydney recommended a triple therapy containing either TDB or bismuth subsalicylate one tablet q.d.s., tetracycline hydrochloride 500 mg q.d.s. and metronidazole 400 mg t.d.s. for 2 weeks. Amoxycillin 500

mg q.d.s. could be used instead of tetracycline but was not as well tolerated [16].

By 1992 Chiba *et al.* [70]were able to publish a meta-analysis showing an eradication rate of 94% in 203 patients treated with these doses of bismuth, tetracycline and metronidazole for 2 weeks (BTM2) and an eradication rate of 73% in 130 patients who received the version with amoxycillin (BAM2). Most of the studies gave results quite close to these figures. The difference is quite convincing, so there is no particular reason to use BAM2, unless the patients is allergic to tetracycline. The main problem with BTM2 is that its complexity can cause poor compliance. Therefore it is necessary to spend time motivating each patient and explaining the details of the regimen – taking bismuth 30 min before meals, taking metronidazole with food, etc. Side effects occur in about a third of patients [16]. Therefore it is not surprising that compliance is the main determinant of success [17] (Figure 5.1). Inferior compliance in 'the real world' may explain why the eradication rate was only 63% when the regimen was used in general practice [99] and 63% in a district general hospital [100].

The side effects are largely due to the antibacterials, particularly metronidazole. Many researchers have therefore tested versions in which the antibiotics or the whole regimen is given for less than 2 weeks. Unfortunately, these studies have generally not been randomized to compare different durations of therapy so that it is difficult to draw any conclusions. Eradication rates obtained with the shorter regimens are generally lower, but not drastically so. Noach, Bosma and Tytgat gave the same doses for 1 week (BTM1) to 78 patients and obtained an eradication rate of 74% [101]. Logan tested a short version of BAM in which bismuth and amoxycillin were given for 1 week in the above doses and metronidazole 400 mg was added for the last 3 days at a higher dose of 500 mg five times daily. This gave an eradication rate of 72% in 106 patients [102]. Bell obtained an eradication rate of 68% with this regimen [100], which was actually slightly better than his result with the more prolonged BTM2. This may reflect the advantage of shorter regimens in 'the real world'. However one can't just keep shortening the regimen. The eradication rate was only 46% when Logan gave bismuth and amoxycillin at the above doses and metronidazole 400 mg five times daily, all for only 3 days [103]!

Other bismuth-based triple therapies
The 4-quinolones ofloxacin and oxacillin can give reasonable eradication rates in bismuth-based triple therapies. Eradication rates of

93% and 85% were obtained using TDB with ofloxacin and amoxycillin [84] or metronidazole and oxacillin [104] respectively. A 10-day triple therapy consisting of TDB, tetracycline and clarithromycin gave an indifferent eradication rate of 72% [105].

Conclusions
Some bismuth-based triple therapies, particularly BTM2, give good eradication rates in clinical trials and are relatively inexpensive. The problem is that they are too complex and frequently cause side effects so that compliance is a substantial problem.

Triple therapy including a drug that suppresses acid secretion
Currently, the most promising approach to eradication of *H. pylori* is with an acid suppressor and two antibiotics. This is a rational approach because the main problem in eradicating this bacterium is that most antibiotics do not work well in acid. The advantage of elevating the pH is clearly seen both *in vitro* and in patients. For instance, eradication rates obtained with amoxycillin rise from zero to about 60% when omeprazole is also given. The third agent pre-sumably interacts in one of the ways described in the introduction to dual therapy (see above). In particular, metronidazole, which works relatively well in an acid milieu, may deal with infection in the minority of persons whose acid secretion is not suppressed by conventional doses of acid suppressor. Meanwhile the other anti-bacterial deals with metronidazole-resistant strains of *H. pylori*. This is well illustrated by Bell, who obtained an eradication rate of 75% in metronidazole-resistant strains using omeprazole 40 mg o.d., amoxycillin 500 mg t.d.s. and metronidazole 400 mg t.d.s. for 2 weeks (OAM2), compared with only 33% with 'World Congress' BTM2 [100]. The use of PPIs simplifies the regimen because they are given only once or twice daily. Bismuth is far less convenient be-cause it has to be taken four times daily and 30 min before meals.

Proton pump inhibitor (PPI), amoxycillin and metronidazole
Bell *et al.* have done by far the biggest trial of this regimen. They gave OAM2 to 263 patients and achieved an eradication rate of 89% [100]. It is relevant that the same group only obtained an eradication rate of 63% using BTM2. The simpler regimen may have improved compliance in their district general hospital setting. An important finding by Bell's group is that the same result is obtained if the regimen is only taken for 1 week (OAM1). *H. pylori* was eradicated from 91% of 80 patients who were given this regimen [106]. It does

seem important to give the antibacterials thrice daily in this regimen. An eradication rate of only 79% was obtained when omeprazole 20 mg, amoxycillin 1 g and metronidazole 400 mg were given b.d. for 1 week to 119 DU patients in the MACH 1 study [107].

Proton pump inhibitor (PPI), clarithromycin and metronidazole or tinidazole
This 1-week regimen was developed by Bazzoli. He gave omeprazole 20 mg o.d., tinidazole 500 mg b.d. and clarithromycin 250 mg b.d. for 1 week [1]. The eradication rate was 95% in 65 patients. Note the low dose of clarithromycin. Moayyedi and Axon [108] gave the same regimen, except that their dose of omeprazole was 20 mg b.d. The eradication rate was 94% in 47 patients. There is no reason to think that their results would be different if metronidazole 400 mg t.d.s. were used instead of tinidazole 500 mg b.d. However, the beauty of Bazzoli's regimen is the convenience of having no lunchtime dose. Tinidazole is more expensive than metronidazole in the UK. Fortunately, metronidazole 400 mg b.d. seems to be equally effective. Labenz *et al.* obtained an eradication rate of 95% in 40 dyspeptic patients given omeprazole 20 mg daily, clarithromycin 250 mg b.d. and metronidazole 400 mg b.d. for one week [109]. The MACH 1 study also obtained an eradication rate of 95% when omeprazole 20 mg, metronidazole 400 mg and clarithromycin 250 mg were given b.d. for 1 week to 111 DU patients (OMC2 50) [107].

Other proton pump inhibitor-based triple therapies
Lamouliatte *et al.* [110] obtained an eradication rate of 90% in 20 patients using omeprazole 20 mg o.d. for 14 days with amoxycillin 1 g b.d. and clarithromycin 500 mg t.d.s. for days 1–10. An eradication rate of 96% was obtained when omeprazole 20 mg, amoxycillin 1 g, and clarithromycin 500 mg were given b.d. for 1 week to 110 DU patients in the MACH 1 study (OAC500). However the eradication rate fell to 84% when the dose of clarithromycin was reduced to 250 mg b.d. [107]. McCarthy *et al.* [111] obtained an eradication rate of only 58% in 43 patients treated for 4 weeks with omeprazole 20 mg o.d., and for one week with metronidazole 400 mg t.d.s. and tetracycline 500 mg t.d.s. Interestingly amoxycillin seems better than tetracycline in triple therapy with omeprazole, while the reverse is true in bismuth-based triple regimens.

Histamine H_2-receptor antagonist with two antibacterials
The largest and best known of these studies was performed by Hentschel *et al.* in Austria [10] and published in 1993. The regimen

has since been licensed for use in the UK although for a different treatment period than that used in Hentschel's study. Hentschel *et al.* gave ranitidine 300 mg *nocte* for 6 weeks with metronidazole 500 mg t.d.s. and amoxycillin 750 mg t.d.s. for 12 days. The eradication rate was 89%. One unusual aspect of this study was that the rate of metronidazole resistance was only 11%, compared with 28% elsewhere in Europe and 65% in our clinic! Grigoriev *et al.* [104] obtained an eradication rate of 63% using the same drugs but their doses of metronidazole and amoxycillin were both 500 mg b.d. and lower than Hentschel's. In general one would expect the efficacy of regimens based on suppression of acid to depend on how strongly acid secretion is suppressed. Since PPIs are more potent than H_2-antagonists in this respect one would predict that they will prove to be superior in eradication therapy.

Comment
The short, low-dose triple therapies OAM1 and OCT or OCM1 are currently the most attractive regimens for treatment of *H. pylori*. Of these OAM1 is probably less toxic and certainly less expensive. Large randomized trials are now needed to compare these excellent regimens.

Quadruple therapies

Several quadruple therapies have been described but are now re-garded as unnecessarily complex. The complexity of the regimen may impair compliance so that the extra drug does not improve the result. For example Borody, who achieved an eradication rate of 96% with standard BTM2, 'only' obtained an eradication rate of 90% when famotidine was added to a very similar regimen [112]. The same regimen given with omeprazole 20 mg b.d. instead of famotidine gave an eradication rate of 97% [113]. The other large study of quad-ruple therapy was by Thijs, Van Zwet and Moden [105], who obtained an eradication rate of 93% using a similar regimen with famotidine.

SIDE EFFECTS

It is generally unsatisfactory to compare side effect rates between studies from different centres. This is partly because the answer depends on how the question is asked, and partly because different populations are more or less stoical. Therefore the data from Ipswich are particularly useful (see below).

CURRENT CHOICE OF ERADICATION REGIMEN

The Ipswich data are also useful in this respect. On the down side the trials have been performed over several years in a non-randomized fashion. However, these data have the advantage of having been obtained from a UK population in a District General Hospital with our own drug formulations and with eradication diagnosed by urea breath test. The results are summarized in Table 5.2. Small differences in eradication rates should be ignored because true differences cannot be detected without randomizing the patients.

Table 5.2 Non-randomized comparison of regimens by Dr Bell, Ipswich (Costs are taken from the *British National Formulary*, September 1994; calculations assume, perhaps incorrectly, that exactly the required number of tablets or capsules can be prescribed – for example a pack containing 7×40 mg of omeprazole is currently only available in hospitals) CBS = colloidal bismuth subcitrate, O = omeprazole, A = amoxycillin, M = metronidazole, R = ranitidine, C = clarithromycin

Name and composition	% with any side effect	eradication metronidazole			cost (£)
		sens.	res.	overall	
Standard triple therapy ($n = 263$)* CBS 120×4, T 500×4 & M 400×3; 2/52	53	90	33	63	18.41
Borody's triple therapy ($n = 26$)* CBS 120×4, T 500×4, M 200×4; 2/52	48	89	—		17.71
Logan's triple therapy ($n = 28$)* CBS 120×4 & A 500×4; 1/52 M 400×5; last 5 days	48	68	—		10.93
OAM2 ($n = 306$)[†] O 40×1, A 500×3 & M 400×3; 2/52	52	98	76	90	41.97
RAM2 ($n = 48$)[†] R 300×1, A 500×3 & M 400×3; 2/52	59	96	50	75	18.63
OA2 ($n = 67$)* O 40×1 & A 500×3; 2/52	12	48	48	48	39.87
OAM1 ($n = 80$)[‡] O 40×1, A 500×3 & M 400×3; 1/52	33	93	88	91	20.98
OCM1 ($n = 118$)[¶] O 40×1, C 250×3 & M 400×3; 1/52	37	97	56	86	35.30

* = [100], [†] = [115] (submitted to *Q J Med*), [‡] = [116], [¶] = Bell, personal communication

Of the various regimens Bell currently recommends OAM1. In studies there seems to be little or no loss when this is given for 1 week. The results are also similar to those obtained with the more expensive OCM1 regimen. A further consideration is that, if the treatment fails, OCM may leave the patient with strain that is resistant to metronidazole and clarithromycin, while bacteria remaining after OAM will only be resistant to metronidazole. This leaves amoxycillin and clarithromycin free for use in patients who fail to eradicate on OAM1. Bell (personal communication) obtains an eradication rate of > 90% in these patients using omeprazole 40 mg o.d., amoxycillin 500 mg t.d.s. and clarithromycin 250 mg t.d.s. for 2 weeks. On the other hand, in the recently published MACH 1 study, two twice-daily one-week triple regimens, OMC250 and OAC500 (see above) give eradication rates of 95% and 96% respectively in large groups of DU patients, and these are the current favourites. Of these OMC250 is cheaper but OAC500 may be a better choice in regions with much metronidazole resistance.

REFERENCES

1. Bazzoli F, Zagari RM, Fossi S *et al.* Short-term, low-dose triple therapy for eradication of *Helicobacter pylori. Eur J Gastroenterol Hepatol* 1994; **6**: 773–777.
2. Gough KR, Korman MG, Bardhan KD *et al.* Ranitidine and cimetidine in prevention of duodenal ulcer relapse. A double-blind, randomised, multicentre, comparative trial. *Lancet* 1984; **ii**: 659–662.
3. Graham DY, Lew GM, Klein PD *et al.* Effect of treatment of *Helicobacter pylori* infection on the long-term recurrence of gastric or duodenal ulcer. A randomized, controlled study. *Ann Intern Med* 1992; **116**: 705–708.
4. Sarosiek J, Roche JK, Marshall B, McCallum RW. Urease enzyme inhibition by bismuth subsalicylate; a putative antibacterial mechanism. *Gastroenterology* 1990; **98**: A119.
5. Nagata K, Satoh H, Iwahi T *et al.* Potent inhibitory action of the gastric proton pump inhibitor lansoprazole against urease activity of *Helicobacter pylori*: unique action selective for *H. pylori* cells. *Antimicrob Agents Chemother* 1993; **37**: 769–774.
6. Logan RPH, Walker MM, Misiewicz JJ *et al.* Changes in the intragastric distribution of *Helicobacter pylori* during treatment with omeprazole. *Gut* 1995; **36**: 12–16.

7. Ferguson DA, Jr., Li C, Patel NR, Mayberry WR, Chi DS, Thomas E. Isolation of *Helicobacter pylori* from saliva. *J Clin Microbiol* 1993; **31**: 2802–2804.

8. Gavey CJ, Szeto ML, Nwokolo CU *et al.* Bismuth accumulates in the body during treatment with tripotassium dicitrato bismuthate. *Aliment Pharmacol Ther* 1989; **3**: 21–28.

9. Marshall BJ, Goodwin CS, Warren JR *et al.* Prospective double-blind trial of duodenal ulcer relapse after eradication of *Campylobacter pylori. Lancet* 1988; **ii**: 1437–1442.

10. Hentschel E, Brandstatter G, Dragosics B *et al.* Effect of ranitidine and amoxicillin plus metronidazole on the eradication of *Helicobacter pylori* and the recurrence of duodenal ulcer. *N Engl J Med* 1993; **328**: 308–312.

11. Parsonnet J, Blaser MJ, Perez Perez GI *et al.* Symptoms and risk factors of *Helicobacter pylori* infection in a cohort of epidemiologists. *Gastroenterology* 1992; **102**: 41–46.

12. Kuipers EJ, Pena AS, Van Kamp G *et al.* Seroconversion for *Helicobacter pylori. Lancet* 1993; **342**: 328–331.

13. Atherton JC, Spiller RC. The urea breath test for *Helicobacter pylori. Gut* 1994; **35**: 723–725.

14. Kosunen TU, Seppala K, Sarna S, Sipponen P. Diagnostic value of decreasing IgG, IgA, and IgM antibody titres after eradication of *Helicobacter pylori. Lancet* 1992; **339**: 893–895.

15. Hirschl AM, Brandstatter G, Dragosics B *et al.* Kinetics of specific IgG antibodies for monitoring the effect of anti-*Helicobacter pylori* chemotherapy. *J Infect Dis* 1993; **168**: 763–766.

16. Tytgat GNJ, Axon ATR, Dixon MF *et al. Helicobacter pylori*: causal agent in peptic ulcer disease? In: Anonymous, ed. *Working Party Reports.* Melbourne: Blackwell Scientific Publications, 1990: 36–45.

17. Graham DY, Lew GM, Malaty HM *et al.* Factors influencing the eradication of *Helicobacter pylori* with triple therapy. *Gastroenterology* 1992; **102**: 493–496.

18. Labenz J, Leverkus F, Madeya S *et al.* Omeprazole plus amoxycillin for cure of *H. pylori* infection: factors influencing the treatment success (abstract). *Scand J Gastroenterol* 1994; **29**: 1070–1075.

19. Harries AD, Stewart M, Deegan KM *et al. Helicobacter pylori* in Malawi, central Africa. *J Infect* 1992; **24**: 269–276.

20. Anonymous. Results of a multicentre European survey in 1991 of metronidazole resistance in *Helicobacter pylori*. European

Study Group on Antibiotic Susceptibility of *Helicobacter pylori*. *Eur J Clin Microbiol Infect Dis* 1992; **11**: 777–781.

21. Logan RP, Gummett PA, Misiewicz JJ *et al*. One week's anti-*Helicobacter pylori* treatment for duodenal ulcer. *Gut* 1994; **35**: 15–18.

22. Logan RP, Gummett PA, Schaufelberger HD *et al*. Eradication of *Helicobacter pylori* with clarithromycin and omeprazole. *Gut* 1994; **35**: 323–326.

23. Peterson WL, Graham DY, Marshall B *et al*. Clarithromycin as monotherapy for eradication of *Helicobacter pylori*: a randomized, double-blind trial. *Am J Gastroenterol* 1993; **88**: 1860–1864.

24. Rautelin H, Tee W, Seppala K, Kosunen TU. Ribotyping patterns and emergence of metronidazole resistance in paired clinical samples of *Helicobacter pylori*. *J Clin Microbiol* 1994; **32**: 1079–1082.

25. Savarino V, Mela GS, Zentilin P *et al*. Variability in individual response to various doses of omeprazole. Implications for antiulcer therapy. *Dig Dis Sci* 1994; **39**: 161–168.

26. Andersson T, Cederberg C, Edvardsson G *et al*. Effect of omeprazole treatment on diazepam plasma levels in slow versus normal rapid metabolizers of omeprazole. *Clin Pharmacol Ther* 1990; **47**: 79–85.

27. Lind T, Cederberg C, Ekenved G *et al*. Effect of omeprazole – a gastric proton pump inhibitor – on pentagastrin stimulated acid secretion in man. *Gut* 1983; **24**: 270–276.

28. Anonymous. Metronidazole. In: Dollery CT, ed. *Therapeutic drugs*. Edinburgh: Churchill Livingstone, 1991: M170–M176.

29. De Giacomo C, Fiocca R, Villani L *et al*. *Helicobacter pylori* infection and chronic gastritis: clinical, serological, and histologic correlations in children treated with amoxicillin and colloidal bismuth subcitrate. *J Pediatr Gastroenterol Nutr* 1990; **11**: 310–316.

30. Mahony MJ, Wyatt JI, Littlewood JM. Management and response to treatment of *Helicobacter pylori* gastritis. *Arch Dis Child* 1992; **67**: 940–943.

31. Israel DM, Hassall E. Treatment and long-term follow-up of *Helicobacter pylori*-associated duodenal ulcer disease in children. *J Pediatr* 1993; **123**: 53–58.

32. Atherton JC, Cockayne A, Balsitis M *et al*. Detection of the intragastric sites at which *Helicobacter pylori* evades treatment with amoxycillin and cimetidine. *Gut* 1995; **36**: 670–4

33. Cooreman MP, Krausgrill P, Hengels KJ. Local gastric and serum amoxicillin concentrations after different oral application forms. *Antimicrob Agents Chemother* 1993; **37**: 1506–1509.

34. Desai HG, Gill HH, Shankaran K *et al*. Dental plaque: a permanent reservoir of *Helicobacter pylori*? *Scand J Gastroenterol* 1991; **26**: 1205–1208.

35. De Cothi GA, Newbold KM, O'Connor HJ. *Campylobacter*-like organisms and heterotopic gastric mucosa in Meckel's diverticula. *J Clin Pathol* 1989; **42**: 132–134.

36. Dye KR, Marshall BJ, Frierson HF Jr *et al*. *Campylobacter pylori* colonizing heterotopic gastric tissue in the rectum. *Am J Clin Pathol* 1990; **93**: 144–147.

37. Atherton JC, Cullun DJE, Hawkey CJ, Spiller RC. Enhanced eradication of *Helicobacter pylori* by pre- versus postprandial amoxycillin suspension with omeprazole: implications for mode of action (abstract). *Gastroenterology* 1994; **106**: A41

38. Atherton JC, Hudson N, Kirk GE *et al*. Amoxycillin capsules with omeprazole for the eradication of *Helicobacter pylori*. Assessment of the importance of antibiotic dose timing in relation to meals. *Aliment Pharmacol Ther* 1994; **8**: 495–498.

39. Weil J, Bell GD, Powell K *et al*. *Helicobacter pylori*: treatment with combinations of pivampicillin and tripotassium dicitrato bismuthate. *Aliment Pharmacol Ther* 1991; **5**: 543–547.

40. Harris A, Misiewicz JJ. Eradication of *H. pylori*. In: Calam J, ed. *Baillière's Clinical Gastroenterology: Helicobacter pylori*. London: Baillière Tindall, 1995: **9**: 583–613.

41. Prewett EJ, Luk YW, Fraser AG *et al*. Comparison of one-day oral dosing with three bismuth compounds for the suppression of *Helicobacter pylori* assessed by the ^{13}C-urea breath test. *Aliment Pharmacol Ther* 1992; **6**: 97–102.

42. Gorbach SL. Bismuth therapy in gastrointestinal diseases. *Gastroenterology* 1990; **99**: 863–875.

43. Wagstaff AJ, Benfield P, Monk JP. Colloidal bismuth subcitrate. A review of its pharmacodynamic and pharmacokinetic properties, and its therapeutic use in peptic ulcer disease. *Drugs* 1988; **36**: 132–157.

44. Tytgat GN. Bismuth is better. *Scand J Gastroenterol Suppl* 1988; **155**: 16–17.

45. Baron JH, Barr J, Batten J *et al*. Acid, pepsin, and mucus secretion in patients with gastric and duodenal ulcer before and after colloidal bismuth subcitrate (De-Nol). *Gut* 1986; **27**: 486–490.

46. De Beaux AC, Defize J, Hunt RH. The effect of tripotassium dicitrato bismuthate on pepsin activity. *Aliment Pharmacol Ther* 1989; **3**: 381–385.

47. Moshal MG, Gregory MA, Pillay C, Spitaels JM. Does the duodenal cell ever return to normal? A comparison between treatment with cimetidine and DeNol. *Scand J Gastroenterol Suppl* 1979; **54**: 48–51.

48. Martin DF, Hollanders D, May SJ *et al*. Difference in relapse rates of duodenal ulcer after healing with cimetidine or tripotassium dicitrato bismuthate. *Lancet* 1981; **i**: 7–10.

49. Lane MR, Lee SP. Recurrence of duodenal ulcer after medical treatment [published erratum appears in *Lancet* 1988; **ii**: 118]. *Lancet* 1988; **i**: 1147–1149.

50. Axon AT. *Campylobacter pylori* – therapy review. *Scand J Gastroenterol Suppl* 1989; **160**: 35–38.

51. Nwokolo CU, Prewett EJ, Sawyerr AM *et al*. The effect of histamine H2-receptor blockade on bismuth absorption from three ulcer-healing compounds. *Gastroenterology* 1991; **101**: 889–894.

52. Nwokolo CU, Lewin JF, Hudson M, Pounder RE. Transmucosal penetration of bismuth particles in the human stomach. *Gastroenterology* 1992; **102**: 163–167.

53. Madaus S, Schulte Frohlinde E, Scherer C *et al*. Comparison of plasma bismuth levels after oral dosing with basic bismuth carbonate or tripotassium dicitrato bismuthate [published erratum appears in *Aliment Pharmacol Ther* 1992; **6**: 761]. *Aliment Pharmacol Ther* 1992; **6**: 241–249.

54. Anonymous. Idiosyncratic neurotoxicity: clioquinol and bismuth [editorial]. *Lancet* 1980; **i**: 857–858.

55. Playford RJ, Matthews CH, Campbell MJ *et al*. Bismuth induced encephalopathy caused by tripotassium dicitrato bismuthate in a patient with chronic renal failure. *Gut* 1990; **31**: 359–360.

56. Shamburek RD, Schubert ML. Control of gastric acid secretion. Histamine H2-receptor antagonists and $H^+K(^+)$-ATPase inhibitors. *Gastroenterol Clin N Am* 1992; **21**: 527–550.

57. Lanzon Miller S, Pounder RE, Hamilton MR *et al*. Twenty-four-hour intragastric acidity and plasma gastrin concentration before and during treatment with either ranitidine or omeprazole. *Aliment Pharmacol Ther* 1987; **1**: 239–251.

58. Grayson ML, Eliopoulos GM, Ferraro MJ, Moellering RCJ. Effect of varying pH on the susceptibility of *Campylobacter*

pylori to antimicrobial agents. *Eur J Clin Microbiol Infect Dis* 1989; **8**: 888–889.

59. Goodwin CS and McNulty CAM. Bacteriological and pharmacological basis for the treatment of *Helicobacter pylori* infection. In: Rathbone BJ, Heatley RV, eds. *Helicobacter pylori and gastroduodenal disease*. Oxford: Blackwell Scientific Publications, 1992: 224–231.

60. Marshall BJ, Barrett LJ, Prakash C *et al.* Urea protects *Helicobacter (Campylobacter) pylori* from the bactericidal effect of acid. *Gastroenterology* 1990; **99**: 697–702.

61. Iwahi T, Satoh H, Nakao M *et al.* Lansoprazole, a novel benzimidazole proton pump inhibitor, and its related compounds have selective activity against *Helicobacter pylori. Antimicrob Agents Chemother* 1991; **35**: 490–496.

62. Mauch F, Bode G, Malfertheiner P. Identification and characterization of an ATPase system of *Helicobacter pylori* and the effect of proton pump inhibitors (letter). *Am J Gastroenterol* 1993; **88**: 1801–1802.

63. Sjostrom J-E, Berglund M-L, Fryklund J *et al.* Factors affecting the antibacterial activity of omeprazole and structural analogues *in vitro* (abstract). *Acta Gastroenterol Belg* 1993; **56**(suppl): 144.

64. Wilde MI, McTavish D. Omeprazole. *Drugs* 1994; **48**: 91–132.

65. Loft S, Poulsen HE, Sonne J, Dossing M. Metronidazole clearance: a one-sample method and influencing factors. *Clin Pharmacol Ther* 1988; **43**: 420–428.

66. Van Zanten SJ, Goldie J, Hollingsworth J *et al.* Secretion of intravenously administered antibiotics in gastric juice: implications for management of *Helicobacter pylori. J Clin Pathol* 1992; **45**: 225–227.

67. Goodwin CS, Marshall BJ, Blincow ED *et al.* Prevention of nitroimidazole resistance in *Campylobacter pylori* by coadministration of colloidal bismuth subcitrate: clinical and *in vitro* studies. *J Clin Pathol* 1988; **41**: 207–210.

68. Lacey SL, Moss SF, Taylor GW. Metronidazole uptake by sensitive and resistant isolates of *Helicobacter pylori. J Antimicrob Chemother* 1993; **32**: 393–400.

69. Rauws EA, Langenberg W, Houthoff HJ *et al. Campylobacter pyloridis*-associated chronic active antral gastritis. A prospective study of its prevalence and the effects of antibacterial and antiulcer treatment. *Gastroenterology* 1988; **94**: 33–40.

70. Chiba N, Rao BV, Rademaker JW, Hunt RH. Meta-analysis of the efficacy of antibiotic therapy in eradicating *Helicobacter pylori*. *Am J Gastroenterol* 1992; **87**: 1716–1727.
71. Unge P, Gad A, Erilsson K *et al*. Amoxycillin added to omeprazole prevents ulcer relapse in the treatment of duodenal ulcer patients. *Eur J Gastroenterol Hepatol* 1993; **5**: 325–331.
72. McNulty CA, Dent JC, Ford GA, Wilkinson SP. Inhibitory antimicrobial concentrations against *Campylobacter pylori* in gastric mucosa. *J Antimicrob Chemother* 1988; **22**: 729–738.
73. Ericsson CD, Feldman S, Pickering LK, Cleary TG. Influence of subsalicylate bismuth on absorption of doxycycline. *JAMA* 1982; **247**: 2266–2267.
74. Unge P, Gnarpe H. Pharmacokinetic, bacteriological and clinical aspects on the use of doxycycline in patients with active duodenal ulcer associated with *Campylobacter pylori*. *Scand J Infect Dis Suppl* 1988; **53**: 70–73.
75. Hardy DJ, Hanson CW, Hensey DM *et al*. Susceptibility of *Campylobacter pylori* to macrolides and fluoroquinolones. *J Antimicrob Chemother* 1988; **22**: 631–636.
76. Peters DH, Clissold SP. Clarithromycin. A review of its antimicrobial activity, pharmacokinetic properties and therapeutic potential. *Drugs* 1992; **44**: 117–164.
77. Gustavson LE, Kaiser JF, Mukherjee DX *et al*. Evaluation of the pharmacokinetic drug interactions between clarithromycin and omeprazole (abstract). *Am J Gastroenterol* 1994; **89**: 1373.
78. Graham DY, Opekun AR, Klein PD. Clarithromycin for the eradication of *Helicobacter pylori*. *J Clin Gastroenterol* 1993; **16**: 292–294.
79. Braegger CP, Nadal D. Clarithromycin and pseudomembranous enterocolitis (letter). *Lancet* 1994; **343**: 241–242.
80. Bell DG, Powell KU, Burridge SM *et al*. *Helicobacter pylori* treated with combinations of tripotassium dicitrato bismuthate and metronidazole: Efficacy of different treatment regimes and some observations on the emergence of metronidazole resistance. *Eur J Gastroenterol Hepatol* 1992; **3**: 819–822.
81. De Koster E, Burette A, Nyst JF. *H. pylori* treatment; amoxycillin or bismuth plus nitroimidazole? (abstract). *Gastroenterology* 1991; **100**: A52.
82. Morgando A, Todros L, Boero M *et al*. Therapy of *Helicobacter pylori* infection: clinical trials with double and triple pharmacological association. *Ital J Gastroenterol* 1991; **23**(suppl 2): 112.

83. Grigoriev PV, Ariun LI, Isakov VA. De-Nol plus oxacillin vs. ranitidine and oxacillin in Hp positive duodenal ulcers (abstract). *Rev Espan Enferm Dig* 1990; **78**(suppl 1): 129.

84. Peyre S, Bologna E, Stroppiana M *et al.* Eradication rate of *Helicobacter pylori* with 4 different regimes (abstract). *Rev Espan Enferm Dig* 1990; **78**(suppl 1): 107–108.

85. Rosario M, Alves I, Martins F *et al.* Combination of bismuth subcitrate and furazolidone in eradication therapy (abstract). *Gastroenterology* 1992; **102**: A45.

86. Tuo BG, Li YN, Ye SM. The efficacy of colloidal bismuth subcitrate and furazolidone on *Helicobacter pylori* (abstract). *Eur J Gastroenterol Hepatol* 1993; **8**(suppl 2): S199.

87. Logan RPH, Rubio MA, Gummett PA. Omeprazole and amoxycillin suspension for *Helicobacter pylori* (abstract). *Irish J Med Sci* 1992; **161**(suppl 10): 16.

88. Labenz J, Stolte M, Domain C *et al.* Omeprazole plus amoxycillin or clarithromycin for eradication of Hp in DU disease (abstract). *Acta Gastro-Enterol Belg* 1993; **56**(suppl 131): 139.

89. Mannes GA, Bayerdorffer E, Hele C *et al.* An increasing dose of omeprazole combined with amoxycillin increases the eradication rate of *Helicobacter pylori* (abstract). *Gastroenterology* 1993; **104**: A140.

90. Zala G, Wirth HP, Giezendanner S *et al.* Omeprazole/amoxycillin: Impaired eradication of *H. pylori* by smoking but not by omeprazole pretreatment (abstract). *Gastroenterology* 1994; **106**: A215

91. Katelaris PH, Patchett SE, Zhang ZW *et al.* A randomised prospective comparison of clarithromycin versus amoxycillin in combination with omeprazole for eradication of *Helicobacter pylori Aliment Pharmacol Ther* 1995; **9**: 205–208

92. Schaufelberger HD, Logan HD, Misiewicz JJ *et al.* The dose and frequency of omeprazole are important in treating *H. pylori* with dual therapy (abstract). *Gastroenterology* 1993; **104**: A186.

93. Schaufelberger HD, Logan RPH, Baron JH, Misiewicz JJ. The effect of compliance on *H. pylori* eradication with dual therapy (abstract). *Schweiz Med Wochenschr* 1993; **123**(suppl 55): 21P.

94. Mendleson M, Greaves R, Logan RPH *et al.* Eradication of *H. pylori* with clarithromycin and omeprazole (abstract). *Gut* 1992; **33**(suppl 2): T108.

95. Chen SP, Xiao SD, Hu FL. Combined omeprazole/antibiotic

treatments for eradication of *Helicobacter pylori* in patients with duodenal ulcer – pilot studies. *Eur J Gastroenterol Hepatol* 1993; 8(suppl 2): S265.

96. Marchegiani A, Di Capua F. Combined omeprazole / azithromycin therapy regime for eradication of *Helicobacter pylori*. *Acta Gastro-Enterol Belg* 1993; 56(suppl): 141.
97. Labenz J, Ruhi GH, Domian C *et al*. Omeprazole plus roxythromycin for eradication of *H. pylori*. *Acta Gastro-Enterol Belg* 1993; 56(suppl): 138.
98. Malfertheiner P. Compliance, adverse events and antibiotic resistance in *Helicobacter pylori* treatment. *Scand J Gastroenterol Suppl* 1993; **196**: 34–37.
99. Cottrill MRB. The prevalence of *Helicobacter pylori* infection in patients receiving long-term H_2-receptor antagonists in general practice: clinical and financial consequences of eradication using omeprazole plus amoxycillin or 'triple therapy'. *Br J Med Econ* 1994; **7**: 35–41.
100. Bell GD, Powell KU, Burridge SM *et al*. *Helicobacter pylori* eradication: efficacy and side effect profile of a combination of omeprazole, amoxycillin and metronidazole compared with four alternative regimens. *Q J Med* 1993; **86**: 743–750.
101. Noach LA, Bosma NB, Tytgat GNJ. CBS and clarithromycin: alternative therapy for *Helicobacter pylori* infection in patients with metronidazole resistant strains? (abstract). 2nd United European Gastroenterology Week, Barcelona 1993; A98.
102. Logan RP, Gummett PA, Misiewicz JJ *et al*. One week eradication regimen for *Helicobacter pylori*. *Lancet* 1991; **338**: 1249–1252.
103. Logan RPH, Gummett RA, Walker MM *et al*. A three-day eradication regime for *Helicobacter pylori* (abstract). *Ital J Gastroenterol* 1991; **23**(suppl 2): 111.
104. Grigoriev PY, Isakov VA, Yakovenko EP, Yakovenko AV. Two different triple therapy regimes for Hp positive duodenal ulcers (abstract). *Ital J Gastroenterol* 1991; **23**(suppl 2): 107–108.
105. Thijs JC, Van Zwet AA, Moden W *et al*. Short report: Clarithromycin, an alternative to metronidazole in the triple therapy of *Helicobacter pylori* infection. *Aliment Pharmacol Ther* 1994; **8**: 131–4
106. Bell DG, Powell KU, Burridge SM *et al*. Rapid eradication of *Helicobacter pylori* infection. *Aliment Pharmacol Ther* 1995; **9**: 41–46.
107. Lind T, Veldhuywen van Zanten SJO, Unge P *et al*. The MACH 1 study: optimal one-week treatment for *H. pylori* is defined? *Gut* 1995; **37** (Suppl 1): A4.

108. Moayyedi P, Axon ATR. Efficacy of a new one week triple therapy regime in eradicating *Helicobacter pylori* (abstract). *Gut* 1994; **35**(suppl 1): F248.

109. Labenz J, Stolte M, Ruhl GH *et al*. One-week low-dose triple therapy for eradication of *Helicobacter pylori* infection. *Eur J Gastroenterol Hepatol* 1995; **7**: 9–11.

110. Lamouliatte H, Cayla R, Zerbib F, Megraud F. Dual therapy versus triple therapy of *Helicobacter pylori* eradication (abstract). *Gastroenterology* 1994; **106**: A120.

111. McCarthy CJ, Collins R, Beattie S *et al*. Short report: treatment of *Helicobacter pylori*-associated duodenal ulcer with omeprazole plus antibiotics. *Aliment Pharmacol Ther* 1993; **7**: 463–466.

112. Borody T, Andrews P, Brandl S, Devine M. *H. pylori* eradication, side effects compliance: 14 days vs 12 day triple therapy. *Gastroenterology* 1993; **104**: A44.

113. Borody TJ, Andrews P, Shortis NP *et al*. Optimal *H. pylori* therapy – a combination of omeprazole and triple therapy (abstract). *Gastroenterology* 1994; **106**: A55.

114. Malanoski GJ, Eliopoulos GM, Ferraro MJ, Moellering RCJ. Effect of pH variation on the susceptibility of *Helicobacter pylori* to three macrolide antimicrobial agents and temafloxacin. *Eur J Clin Microbiol Infect Dis* 1993; **12**: 131–133.

115. Powell KU, Bell GD, Bowden A *et al*. *Helicobacter pylori* eradication therapy: a comparison between either omeprazole or ranitidine in combination with amoxycillin plus metronidazole (abstract). *Gut* 1994; **35**(suppl 5): S16.

116. Bell DG, Powell KU, Burridge SM *et al*. Rapid eradication of *Helicobacter pylori* infection. *Aliment Pharmacol Ther* 1995; **9**: 41–46

6

Management strategies

INTRODUCTION

The discovery that several common gastroduodenal diseases are largely due to a bacterium which is relatively easy to diagnose and treat has called for a complete re-think of our clinical strategies. This chapter will explore the new possibilities and how they can be realized. Of course, the scene is constantly changing and current flow-charts may soon be history. The list of indications for eradication therapy is likely to lengthen. Family practitioners are likely to play a greater role as diagnostic kits improve and eradication regimens are rationalized. New approaches might decrease the load on overstretched endoscopy services, but if so it will be especially important to maintain a rigorous attitude to potentially serious conditions. Gastric cancer is now a curable disease if it is diagnosed early enough. Of patients undergoing curative resection of early gastric cancer, 60% survived for 5 years in Leeds [1]. A study in Birmingham showed that early endoscopy increases the chance of finding these early lesions [2]. I will discuss the possibilities by considering some of the commoner clinical scenarios.

PATIENTS WHOSE GASTROINTESTINAL DIAGNOSIS IS KNOWN

A patient with a duodenal ulcer (Figure 6.1)

It is now clear that these patients should have *H. pylori* eradicated. This was agreed by the NIH consensus meeting in 1994 [3]. Eradication permanently cures the condition in the great majority of patients, and prevents life-threatening complications such as haemorrhage (Chapter 3). We are left discussing the details.

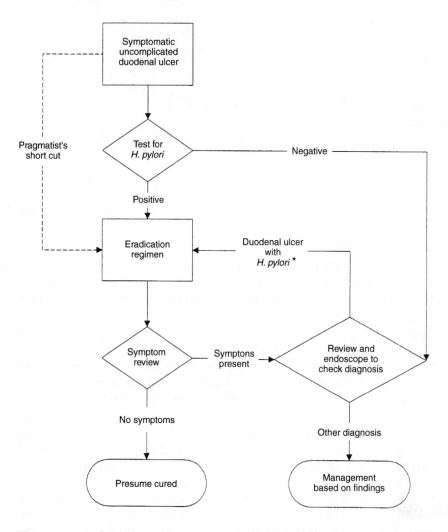

Figure 6.1 A flow chart for management of a patient with an uncomplicated duodenal ulcer that has been diagnosed without determining the patient's *H. pylori* status. * indicates that the previous test for *H. pylori* gave a false-negative result.

Should the patients be tested for infection before eradication therapy is prescribed?
Good medical practice dictates that infection should be diagnosed before it is treated. Most ulcers are diagnosed by endoscopy and patients can easily be tested for *H. pylori* during the examination. The question of whether to test arises if a definite duodenal ulcer

has been seen either on barium X-ray or by endoscopy in a unit that did not look for the infection.

There are advantages in testing the patient, and this should be done if possible. Unnecessary treatment, its complications and the chance of generating antibiotic-resistant bacteria might be avoided (Chapter 5). The bacterium's sensitivity to antibiotics can be determined (Chapter 4). In addition, the small minority of patients whose DU is not due to *H. pylori* can be identified and other causes, such as the use of NSAIDs, Crohn's disease or the Zollinger–Ellison syndrome, can be diagnosed. Patients may be more motivated to take their treatment if they know that they are definitely rather than probably infected.

Despite this, it might sometimes be reasonable to treat without testing, for instance in a general practice where tests are not readily available. If there is a definite duodenal ulcer the chance of infection being present is greater than the sensitivity of many of the tests (Chapter 3). It is not obligatory to determine whether the patient's strain is resistant to metronidazole because modern regimes such as 'OAM' eradicate about 75% of metronidazole-resistant strains [4]. The patients whose DU is not due to *H. pylori* will return with persistent symptoms soon enough! The patient should of course be re-endoscoped anyway if the pattern of symptoms changes.

Hopefully in future technical improvements and different financial arrangements will allow us all to diagnose this infection properly before reaching for the prescription pad!

Is it necessary to heal the ulcer before prescribing eradication therapy?
The short answer is no. The idea of delaying eradication is a hangover from a phase when eradication therapy was mistakenly reserved for patients with persistent or recurrent ulcers. There is no point in delaying therapy which will permanently cure the patient's disease. In addition, successful eradication heals a higher percentage of ulcers compared with simple suppression of acid secretion, at least if this is with an H_2-antagonist [5]. Another reason for starting with eradication therapy comes from studies showing that omeprazole and amoxycillin is less effective if it is given to a patient who is already on omeprazole [6]. The idea is that omeprazole puts *H. pylori* bacteria into a state that is less susceptible to antibiotics. It is not clear whether triple therapies are also susceptible to this problem.

Of course, there are some clinical situations in which ulcer-healing therapy is likely to be given first, such as when illness makes the patient unable to take the antibacterials or to keep them down!

Intravenous eradication therapy is possible [7] but no more effective. Therefore it is generally better to wait until the patient can take less expensive medication by mouth.

Is it necessary to continue the ulcer-healing therapy when treating an active ulcer with eradication therapy?
It is not clear whether a patient with an active ulcer who has received 1-week triple therapy, for example, benefits from continuing the ulcer-healing element after the week has passed. DU disease is by nature cyclical and ulcers tend to heal spontaneously. It is certainly advisable to continue therapy until eradication has been confirmed if the patient has suffered a serious complication such as haemorrhage (Figure 6.2).

Is it necessary to re-test the patient after therapy?
Re-testing provides the advantage of reassuring the patient and doctor that the job has been completed. Persisting infection can be diagnosed and treated without the patient having to endure a further exacerbation. It is generally agreed that patients who have bled should be re-tested before stopping maintenance therapy (Figure 6.2). Unfortunately re-testing currently requires endoscopy or a breath test 1–2 months after the end of eradication therapy. Breath testing is not widely available nationwide and waiting lists for endoscopy are generally long. Therefore I do not regard re-testing as mandatory in patients who have had an uncomplicated duodenal ulcer. Of course, if patients are not re-tested they should be warned that the ulcer might recur.

What should we do with the patient who returns with symptoms after a single attempt at eradication therapy?
A minimalist approach is only acceptable if the patient is doing well. Patients who return with symptoms should be investigated by endoscopy. The aims at this stage are to obtain an accurate diagnosis, to establish whether *H. pylori* is present and if so, which antibiotics it is sensitive to. The urgency depends on clinical circumstances and a patient with symptoms on a long waiting list can be given alkalis, but treatments likely to produce false-negative endoscopy results should be avoided.

The patient with a chronic gastric ulcer (Figure 6.3)

About 70% of these patients are infected with *H. pylori*. In that case the chance of ulcer recurrence and of complications such as

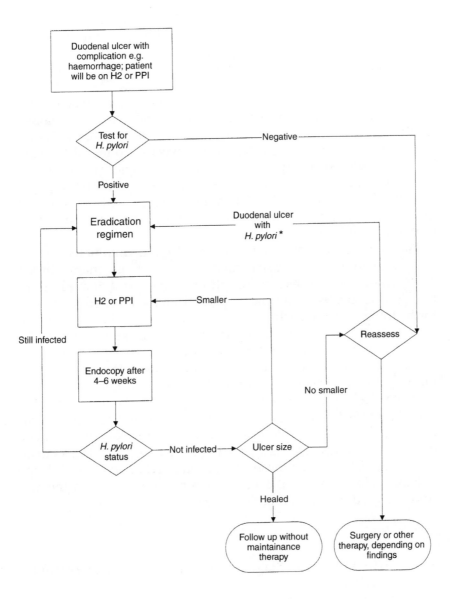

Figure 6.2 A flow chart for management of a patient with a duodenal ulcer with a complication such as haemorrhage. Surgical advice should be sought if there is a recurrence of the complication, such as a re-bleed, at any time. H2 = histamine H2-receptor antagonist; PPI = proton pump inhibitor. * indicates that the previous test for *H. pylori* gave a false-negative result.

haemorrhage are greatly diminished by eradicating *H. pylori* (Chapter 3). Therefore these patients should be tested for *H. pylori* and treated if it is present. As in the case of DU patients (see above) it could be argued that GU patients should be assumed to be infected, particularly if they are not taking NSAIDs. The arguments for and against testing are similar to those in DU disease (see above), except that GU patients are more likely to give false- negative biopsy results because they usually have extensive gastric atrophy. Therefore, if the patient is to be tested, it is advisable to test at least six biopsies (we use inexpensive 'in-house' biopsy urease tests) (Chapter 4), or to use a non-invasive test. In my view the finding that *H. pylori* is less prevalent in GU than in DU patients (Chapter 3) makes it particularly worthwhile establishing whether the infection is present in this group of patients.

The management of chronic gastric ulcers is dominated by the need to diagnose early gastric cancers or malignant change in the ulcer. These patients need to be endoscoped every 4–6 weeks until the ulcer has healed. Multiple biopsies from the ulcer edge are sent for histology during each examination. Surgery is indicated if the ulcer fails to heal, or if the histological appearances are suspicious. This is the time-honoured approach. However *H. pylori* should now be sought at the first endoscopy and eradicated if it is present. The ulcer-healing drug is then continued with endoscopic surveillance until the ulcer has healed. These patients should be retested after the end of therapy to ensure that the infection has been cured, particularly if the lesion is definitely benign but slow to heal. This could be done by breath test, after transferring the patient for 2 weeks to an H_2-antagonist, because these do not interfere with this test. If the patient remains infected, a further course of eradication therapy could be tried before calling the surgeon.

The patient with a firm diagnosis of gastro-oesophageal reflux disease (GORD).

At the time of writing there is no evidence that these patients benefit from eradication of *H. pylori*, if it is present. Therefore it is currently unnecessary to test them for *H. pylori* infection, or to treat the bacterium if it is present.

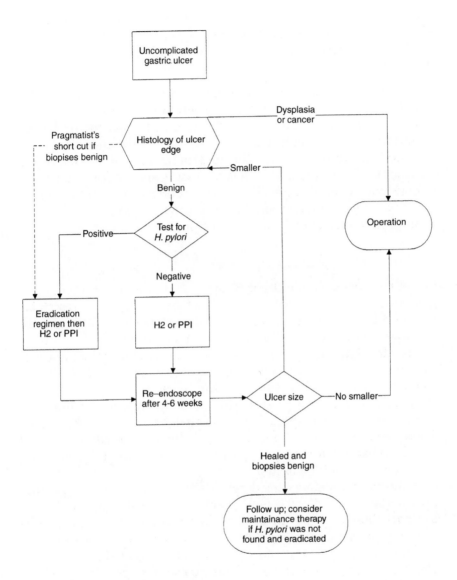

Figure 6.3 A flow chart for management of a patient with an uncomplicated chronic gastric ulcer. H$_2$ = histamine H$_2$-receptor antagonist; PPI = proton pump inhibitor.

The patient has one or more gastric mucosal lesions containing an excess of lymphocytes, prominent lymphoid nodules, a MALT lymphoma or a non-Hodgkin's lymphoma of the stomach

These lesions, particularly the milder ones, may disappear after *H. pylori* is eradicated (Chapter 3). Therefore it is certainly worth testing for the bacterium and eradicating it if it is present, before undertaking more drastic treatment options. Endoscopy should be repeated 1–2 months after the end of treatment to determine whether the infection and the lesions have gone. Follow-up examinations will generally be needed with a frequency depending on the severity of the original lesion. Lesions which progress or recur after healing should obviously be treated along conventional lines.

The patient at risk of gastric cancer

Of course it is useless to treat *H. pylori* in a patient with incurable gastric cancer. These patients have often in any case lost their infection by developing gastric atrophy. However one might ask whether it is worth treating the patient's relatives, or individuals with a strong family history of gastric cancer. The problem here is that there has been no prospective study of whether eradicating *H. pylori* decreases the risk of subsequent cancer. Such trials have been started but it will take several years to see the result. The infection particularly increases the risk of cancer if it is acquired in childhood. Therefore eradication at a young age is likely to lessen the risk of cancer. What we don't know is whether eradicating long-standing infection in adult life has any effect.

In the meantime, since the diagnosis and treatment of *H. pylori* are now relatively simple, it seems reasonable to treat individuals who are particularly at risk of gastric cancer if they are found to be infected, particularly if they are young. This will at least provide reassurance and in this context patients should be re-tested to show that eradication has been successful. *H. pylori* is specifically associated with cancers of the intestinal type. Therefore it would be sensible to eradicate the infection from patients who have had an intestinal-type gastric cancer successfully resected.

The fully investigated non-ulcer dyspeptic

At the time of writing the overall evidence indicates that these patients do not benefit from eradication of *H. pylori*. Therefore it is strictly inappropriate to seek or treat the infection, although in the real world it might be difficult to resist doing so. A small proportion of these patients may have duodenal ulcers which were in the healed phase at the time of investigation. The discovery and eradication of the infection is likely to exert a strong placebo effect. This may be a curse in research but can be a blessing in the clinic! Finally, eradication might prevent the younger patient from developing cancer in later life. Therefore, writing as a clinician rather than a scientist, if I find *H. pylori* **during investigations that have excluded other potential causes of the patient's dyspepsia** I treat it. Fortunately, some large prospective studies are in progress which should help to clarify this rather murky area.

PATIENTS WHOSE GASTROINTESTINAL DIAGNOSIS IS NOT KNOWN

The patient presenting with dyspepsia

Introduction
This is currently the most controversial scenario for a number of reasons.

Patient requirements
- Patients with DUs or GUs, not taking NSAIDs, are almost always infected with *H. pylori*. These patients benefit so much from eradication therapy that they should certainly receive it.
- However DUs and GUs only account for about 10–20% of dyspepsia. Most patients presenting with this symptom have other conditions, including gastro-oesophageal reflux disease (GORD), non-ulcer dyspepsia (NUD) or the irritable bowel syndrome (IBS) [8], which do not appear to benefit from eradication of *H. pylori*.
- Diagnosis of the cause of dyspepsia by history and examination is frequently incorrect [9]. The correct diagnosis can only be arrived at by endoscopy or barium X-ray.
- If gastric cancer is diagnosed early it can be cured by surgery in about 60% of cases in a good centre [1]. Delay in diagnosis diminishes the chance of finding early tumours [2]. The following features are particularly suggestive of gastric cancer:
  – new dyspepsia over the age of 40 years;
  – anorexia;

- weight loss;
- family history of gastric cancer.
- Eradication of *H. pylori* might decrease the risk of gastric cancer in later life, particularly if the treatment is given at a young age. However this benefit is not proven.
- *H. pylori* is common in the general population and does not cause disease in most individuals (Chapter 2).

Situations to avoid
- It is undesirable to give eradication therapy to patients who will not benefit from it because:
  - patients are subjected to unnecessary risk and side effects;
  - the doctor–patient relationship is harmed by lack of response;
  - money is wasted.
- It is particularly bad to give eradication therapy to patients who are not infected!
- A course of treatment which includes metronidazole but does not eradicate *H. pylori* is very likely to produce metronidazole-resistant strains (Chapter 5), and should therefore be avoided.

Cost-efficiency
- Gastric cancer is rare under the age of 45 years. A study of 1153 patients undergoing endoscopy in Leeds asked what would happen if the examination was not done in patients who are:
  - not taking NSAIDs;
  - negative on serological testing for *H. pylori*;
  - under 45 years old [10].

  Serology may be particularly suitable for this approach because, unlike the urea breath test, it indicates past infection and is not altered by recent therapy. This policy would have avoided endoscopy in 265 patients, thus diminishing their endoscopic workload by 23%. They would have missed six peptic ulcers but no malignant lesions. Of course, one has to accept that malignant lesions in young people would eventually be missed if such a policy were applied. The question is whether shortening the waiting list in a particular practice would help more patients than it harms.

Lack of resources for optimal management
- **In hospital**: Most endoscopy waiting-lists are too long. This can lead to two problems:
  - gastric cancer is usually not diagnosed until after it has become unresectable;

- how should we treat dyspepsia while the patient waits for endoscopy?
- **In general practice**: *H. pylori* can be diagnosed by breath test or serology in general practice, but the resources and arrangements for this are generally not in place.

Clinical strategy (Figure 6.4)

This section becomes more controversial as it proceeds and it is essential that strategies are agreed locally between general practitioners and gastroenterologists.

'New' dyspepsia over the age of 45 years

Patients presenting with dyspepsia for the first time, or with a change in the nature of their symptoms when over the age of 45 years, should be endoscoped promptly to exclude early gastric cancer. There should be a 'fast-track' for these patients [2]. Patients are most likely to have gastric cancer if they have alarming symptoms such as anorexia or weight loss, but all patients in this group should be examined promptly because early gastric cancer does not always present with this typical picture. Management after endoscopy depends on what is found.

Dyspepsia under the age of 45 years

A policy is emerging for younger dyspeptics based on initial non-invasive diagnosis of their *H. pylori* status.

Uninfected dyspeptics under 45

Research has indicated a new way of dealing with this group which seems sensible but remains somewhat controversial. If testing indicates that the patient is not infected with *H. pylori* he or she can be treated on the basis of symptoms using antacids, H_2-antagonists or omeprazole in the confidence that no serious lesion is present, except for oesophagitis. It is estimated that about a quarter of endoscopies can be avoided by this policy (see above). Of course, such patients need careful follow up and should be endoscoped promptly if progress is unsatisfactory.

Infected under-45-year-olds

Here the policy becomes even more controversial. The choice of approach depends on the local situation.

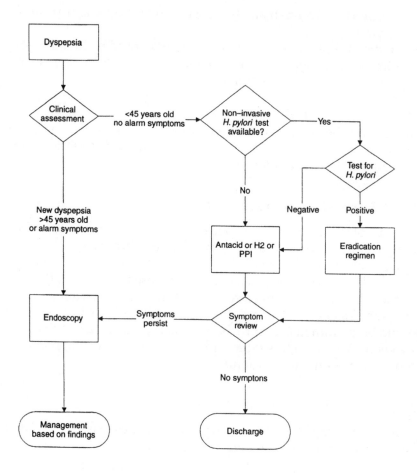

Figure 6.4 A flow chart for management of a patient presenting with dyspepsia of unknown cause which has failed to respond to lifestyle measures and antacids. H_2 = histamine H_2-receptor antagonist; PPI = proton pump inhibitor.

Endoscopy first

The advantage of endoscoping these patients is that a precise diagnosis is obtained at the start. Eradication therapy is reserved for ulcer patients who will definitely benefit. This avoids the expense and risk of giving eradication therapy to non-ulcer patients in whom an advantage has not been established. The main argument against this approach emanates from the expense and risk associated with endoscopy. In addition, if it turns out that eradicating *H. pylori* from under-40-year-olds does decrease their risk of cancer, then the non-ulcer patients will not have received this benefit. With this policy it is important that therapy given in the interim does not render the endoscopy useless, either by healing lesions or by making the bacterium undetectable.

Eradication therapy first
This approach will heal the peptic ulcers, avoid the expense, etc. of endoscopy and might protect the patient from cancer in later life. On the other hand, the widespread use of eradication therapy in this group will produce unnecessary side effects and may lead to the emergence of resistant strains. In addition, most of the current evidence suggests that the majority of the patients who receive eradication therapy will not gain symptomatic relief from it, except perhaps through a placebo effect (Chapter 3).

Which one?
The central ethos of diagnosis before treatment demands endoscopy first but in the real world a trial of eradication therapy has much to commend it.

REFERENCES

1. Sue Ling HM, Johnston D, Martin IG *et al*. Gastric cancer: a curable disease in Britain. *Br Med J* 1993; **307**: 591–596.
2. Hallissey MT, Allum WH, Jewkes AJ *et al*. Early detection of gastric cancer. *Br Med J* 1990; **301**: 513–515.
3. Anonymous. NIH Consensus Conference. *Helicobacter pylori* in peptic ulcer disease. NIH Consensus Development Panel on *Helicobacter pylori* in Peptic Ulcer Disease. *JAMA* 1994; **272**: 65–69.
4. Bell GD, Powell KU, Burridge SM *et al*. *Helicobacter pylori* eradication: efficacy and side effect profile of a combination of omeprazole, amoxycillin and metronidazole compared with four alternative regimens. *Q J Med* 1993; **86**: 743–750.
5. Marshall BJ, Goodwin CS, Warren JR *et al*. Prospective double-blind trial of duodenal ulcer relapse after eradication of *Campylobacter pylori*. *Lancet* 1988; **ii**: 1437–1442.
6. Labenz J, Leverkus F, Borsch G. Omeprazole plus amoxycillin for the cure of *Helicobacter pylori* infection: factors affecting treatment success. *Scand J Gastroenterol* 1994; **29**: 1070–1075.
7. Adamek RJ, Wegener M, Labenz J *et al*. Medium-term results of

oral and intravenous omeprazole/amoxicillin *Helicobacter pylori* eradication therapy. *Am J Gastroenterol* 1994; **89**: 39–42.

8. Befrits R, Granstrom M, Rylander M, Rubio C. *Helicobacter pylori* in 205 consecutive endoscopy patients. *Scand J Infect Dis* 1993; **25**: 185–191.

9. Talley NJ, Weaver AL, Tesmer DL, Zinsmeister AR. Lack of discriminant value of dyspepsia subgroups in patients referred for upper endoscopy. *Gastroenterology* 1993; **105**: 1378–1386.

10. Sobala GM, Crabtree JE, Pentith JA *et al.* Screening dyspepsia by serology to *Helicobacter pylori. Lancet* 1991; **338**: 94–96.

7

The future

INTRODUCTION

In the future we can expect to see further improvements in the diagnosis and treatment of *H. pylori*. The infection may eventually be prevented by immunization and hopefully also by improved public health. The indications for treatment in patients without ulcers are likely to expand and become more clearly defined. The new approaches to treatment may change the respective roles of the family practitioner and hospital-based gastroenterologist in the management of upper gastrointestinal diseases. The aim of this chapter is to describe some of the developments that are already underway and to discuss how further advances might come about.

BIOPSY-BASED TESTS

Biochemical testing of biopsies

H. pylori's urease is so potent that it is difficult to imagine any better reaction to base biochemical testing on. The biopsy urease test has not really been developed this decade. We really need the result before patients leave the endoscopy unit. Detection is by change in pH, so the amount of buffering is crucial. The 'one-minute' test contains no buffer [1], but this makes it unstable in storage. We find it necessary to freeze the solution until the day of use, or make it up freshly each day. 'Spontaneous' changes in the pH are presumably due to absorption of atmospheric gasses or bacterial growth. Both these problems are potentially soluble, for example by aliquoting the solution under nitrogen, and under sterile conditions or with an antibacterial agent added.

At the other end of the spectrum, McNulty's robust recipe [2] contains buffer but may take 24 h to give the correct result. Clearly the amount of buffer needs to be optimized. All the current tests use phenol red, which is cheap and changes colour over the range from pH 6.6 to pH 8.0. There is a wide variety of other pH indicators, which change colour at different pH points and should also be considered. One could use an indicator which detects ammonium ions instead of pH, but this might give false-positive results in patients with liver or renal failure. The biopsy urease test can give false-positive results in patients who have other urea-splitting bacteria in neutral gastric juice [3,4]. It might be possible to find conditions or a selective enzyme inhibitor which renders other bacterial ureases inactive. The CLO test contains antibacterial agent to prevent the growth of these bacteria during incubation of the test.

Culture of biopsies

In our experience the main problem here occurs during transport of biopsies to the laboratory. This can be overcome by improving systems within the hospital, and also by better transport media (Chapter 4). *H. pylori* are microaerophilic bacteria which might be damaged by atmospheric oxygen during transport. This problem needs to be defined and addressed. The development of bacterio-logical culture techniques is beyond the scope of this book.

Histology

The detection of *H. pylori* at histology could be improved by im-munological staining or *in situ* PCR but these techniques are expen-sive and time-consuming. Results may be improved more cheaply by careful selection of special stains, as described in Chapter 4.

Sampling

The central problem is that the biopsy forceps may land on an uninfected area of an infected stomach. This problem is greatest with single biopsies, so kits such as the CLO test should be adapted to use at least two biopsies. Also, we need to know more precisely where to take biopsies from in patients who have recently taken proton pump inhibitors. These decrease the number of bacteria in the gastric antrum while bacterial counts in the gastric corpus are unchanged or even increased [5].

There are two other ways to overcome sampling problems at

endoscopy. Firstly, the stomach can be sprayed with an indicator via the endoscope and then inspected. Such an indicator might show where the bacteria are likely to be, for instance where there is no atrophy, to allow a rational choice of biopsy site. Alternatively the indicator could reveal *H. pylori* itself. Kohli *et al.* could detect *H. pylori* by spraying the stomach via the endoscope with 0.05% phenol red and 0.5 M urea [6]. However it was necessary to elevate the intragastric pH to 4.0–5.0 by premedication with a proton pump inhibitor or H_2-antagonist. The problem here is that pH-based testing may give erratic results because the intragastric pH varies so much between patients. Therefore it would be useful to use an indicator of some other product, such as ammonium ions.

Secondly, sampling problems can be overcome by testing gastric juice rather than individual biopsies. PCR of gastric juice detected the bacteria in 96% of infected persons [7]. Development might make this sufficiently sensitive to overcome sampling problems. PCR will become much more specific as primers are chosen more carefully. Rapid PCR kits are technically feasible but one really does have to be exceedingly careful to avoid contaminating samples with DNA from other bacteria. A simpler approach is to test gastric juice for products of *H. pylori*. For instance the infection can be detected by measuring urea and ammonia or the ratio of these in gastric juice [8].

Brushings
Another way to get around the problem of sampling might be to take cytology brushings instead of biopsies. The brush could sample a wider area than biopsy forceps do. The brushings can be stained either with conventional stains [9] or with monoclonal antibodies [10]. However the sensitivity and specificity of this approach remains unclear because of the current lack of adequate standards.

Comment

At present there is a relative lack of interest in developing endoscopy-based tests further, even though the sensitivity of current methods is generally about 90% or less. This is partly justified, because false negatives are often due to the patient being sampled at the wrong time rather than a fault in the test. It certainly is important to avoid sampling patients while they are on treatments. However there is still room for useful innovation in endoscopy-based tests.

NON-INVASIVE TESTS

Serology

We already have kits that show the patient's *H. pylori* status from finger-prick blood within a few minutes. Now we need financial arrangements to allow these to be widely used. In my opinion they should be available on prescription. Fund-holders can budget for them but it may be cheaper to send serum to the hospital for ELISA. Test may soon be sold 'over the counter' but this is not ideal because those most likely to be infected are least able to afford the kits (Chapter 2)!

From the technical point of view the *H. pylori* antigens could be improved by studying the antibodies present in patients who currently give false-negative tests. For instance, we find that patients with gastric atrophy often have lower serum IgG antibodies against a mixture of *H. pylori* antigens [11], but higher IgG antibodies to CagA protein [12] than infected individuals without atrophy. Once the relevant antigen is identified it is quite easy to produce large amounts by recombinant techniques.

The urea breath test

Similarly the main problem with the urea breath test is that it is not generally available, rather than any particular problem with the test. It would be useful if inexpensive detectors of $^{13}CO_2$ or $^{14}CO_2$ were available in hospital clinics. Cheaper machines are being developed, but the price is likely to remain prohibitive for the time being. Details of the test are being optimized. It would be useful to develop a protocol for non-fasted patients for use during the first consultation.

Sampling faeces

It is possible to culture *H. pylori* from stools or to detect it by PCR in this material. There are technical problems, as discussed in Chapter 4. These could be overcome, but clinicians are likely to choose other tests for aesthetic reasons!

H. pylori *products in urine, etc.*

H. pylori may well affect the excretion of certain substances such as ammonium ions in urine but nobody has so far developed a useful urine-based test. Unfortunately, tests that do not selectively sample the stomach are likely to be affected by 'noise' from the vast numbers of bacteria in the colon. Similarly, *H. pylori* probably releases substances into the blood or breath, but detection would have to be highly specific to distinguish these from the products of the colonic flora.

Scanning and spectroscopy

It is now possible to obtain detailed biochemical information on internal organs using positron emission tomography (PET) and particularly magnetic resonance spectroscopy (MRS). Technical developments will probably enable these techniques to detect *H. pylori*, but this might be 'using a sledgehammer to crack a nut'!

The identification of pathogenic strains of H. pylori

Some strains of *H. pylori* are undoubtedly more pathogenic than others (Chapters 1 and 3). These can be identified by serology, or culture or PCR of biopsies, gastric juice or faeces (Chapter 4). Patients with ulcers or cancer have toxigenic strains that possess the gene *cagA* more often than infected individuals who only have gastritis (Chapter 5). Unfortunately some individuals with non-toxigenic strains also develop these conditions, so it is not always particularly useful to know the toxin-status of an individual's bacterium. However in future a more detailed knowledge of pathogenic factors will hopefully allow the disease outcome to be predicted more accurately.

TREATMENT

Development of short triple therapies

The development of 1-week triple therapies is a major advance in eradication therapy. These regimens seem so good that the obvious approach is to try to increase the eradication rate from about 90% to 100%. The possible approaches could be applied to any other regimen.

Compliance

Compliance is likely to improve if dosing is entirely b.d., rather than t.d.s. I believe that we really need a 1-week calendar pack with very clear instructions. The problem for the manufacturer has been that regimens tend to be obsolete before the pack has been approved and launched! In the meantime it might be useful to provide a calendar-type checklist of doses taken. Of course, compliance is also improved by a lack of side effects. Therefore it will be important to determine the side-effect profiles of the different regimens in randomized, double blind studies. The problem of compliance could be eliminated by using depot injections of drugs, but this is unacceptable when side effects are common.

Metronidazole-resistant strains
We are looking for a drug which is as acid-resistant and well-distributed as metronidazole, but to which H. pylori does not become resistant. Clarithromycin has the first two features but not the last. Therefore I would like to know much more about how pH perturbs the effectiveness of antibiotics. Since the pH within the bacterium is close to neutral it is likely that a low pH affects uptake of antibiotics across the plasma membrane. Once the nature of the problem has been defined it might be possible to produce acid-proof 'designer drugs'. At present, this looks like the only approach that will produce effective mono- and dual therapies.

Fast eradication strategies

It is technically possible to eradicate H. pylori very rapidly. Kimura et al. eradicated H. pylori from 24 out of 25 patients in a regimen which only involved giving antibacterial agents for **1 hour**. Side effects only occurred in one patient (diarrhoea) [13]. These Japanese patients were given 30 mg of lansoprazole daily and 18 000 tyrosine units of pronase b.d. for the previous 2 days. Pronase is a proteolytic enzyme, which was used to increase exposure of the bacteria to the antibacterial agents which followed. A balloon was then inflated just beyond the bulb of the duodenum to prevent escape of the treatment. Next, 100 ml of 7% sodium bicarbonate containing 1 g of bismuth subnitrate, amoxycillin 2 g, metronidazole 1 g and pronase 30 mg was instilled into the stomach via a tube. The patient's position was then changed every 15 mins from sitting to supine to prone to right lateral in order to irrigate the entire gastric mucosa! Finally, the solution was sucked out. The main lesson from this is that H. pylori can be eradicated rapidly if drugs are delivered effectively to the relevant sites. This raises the possibility that a one-off oral therapy might be feasible.

Laser

Bown's group have tested photodynamic therapy as a means of eradicating *H. pylori*. This involves getting the bacteria to take up a photosensitizing agent so that they are killed by exposure to light. In an *in vitro* study cultures of *H. pylori* took up an aluminium-containing sensitizer and could then be then killed by red laser light [14]. A slightly higher dose of light at the same wavelength produced light necrosis of rat colon, which then healed to normal mucosa. Technical developments might allow *H. pylori* to be eradicated during a single endoscopy without harming the mucosa. The light could be distributed around the stomach by shining the laser into a transparent balloon. One major problem is that it would be necessary to hit sanctuary sites, such as the duodenal bulb and infected Barrett's oesophagus. This is certainly an ingenious approach which might merit further study *in vivo*.

Prevention and treatment by immunization

As *H. pylori* survives the host's immune response it might seem unlikely that immunization could prevent this infection, but happily this is not the case. Several pharmaceutical companies are working on this project but do not publish their results for obvious reasons. However, Lee's university-based group have shown that immunization is feasible. They asked whether immunization can prevent specific-pathogen-free mice from becoming infected with *H. felis*. These animals were given a sonicated *H. felis* mixed with the adjuvant cholera toxin five times over a period of 54 days. When challenged with *H. felis* 3 days later the percentage of animals that acquired the infection was diminished from 100% to 5% [15]. Subsequent studies have shown that the protection is long-lasting (Lee, personal communication). Interestingly, the immunization of infected animals has also been shown to eradicate the infection – 'immuno-eradication' [16]. This is a promising start and further development is under way. The mice are also protected against *H. felis* if they are immunized with a sonicate of *H. pylori* [16] or with recombinant subunit B of *H. pylori*'s urease [17] instead of the crude sonicate of *H. felis*. Less toxic adjuvants are being developed. A product of *E. coli* – CTB – is as effective as cholera toxin but non-toxic. Alternatively the bacterial product can be genetically engineered to remove its toxicity. Once animal models have been successfully developed, studies could progress to human volunteers. The results are awaited with great interest. Once a vaccine has been developed it is possible to envisage that whole populations could be immunized in childhood. Protection of this sort might be particuarly useful in developing countries, where re-infection rates after conventional eradication therapy are high (Chapter 2). Unfortunately, such countries are likely to be the least able to afford this approach.

Extra-gastrointestinal consequences of *H. pylori* infection

Some very interesting results from St George's Hospital suggest that the effects of chronic *H. pylori* infection extend beyond the gastroin-testinal tract. These are mentioned at this late stage because at the time of writing the data are quite preliminary. The resuts of further studies are currently awaited with interest!

Short stature
Mendall *et al.* found that, after correction for factors such as age, sex, and social class, infected persons were 1.42 cm shorter than unin-fected individuals ($p = 0.039$) [18]. This is plausible, because infec-tion is usually acquired in childhood when gastrointestinal disorders can have a marked effect on growth. *H. pylori* was present in 55% of Parisian children under investigation for the short stature syndrome, compared with 18% of controls [19]. Of course the prob-lem with this sort of work is that it is more or less impossible to be sure that every other factor which affects height has been corrected for. This is necessary before one can conclude that *H. pylori* actually causes the shorter stature.

Ischaemic heart disease
Mendall *et al.* recruited 111 consecutive cases with coronary heart disease from their cardiology clinic and compared them with 74 individuals attending a general practice health screening clinic. All were white men aged 45–65 years. Serology showed that 59% of cases were infected, compared with 39% of controls. The difference was only slightly diminished by correction for social class and childhood environment [20]. They have now shown that individuals infected with *H. pylori* have elevated serum fibrinogen levels [21]. This is interesting because high levels of fibrinogen are accepted to increase the risk of ischaemic heart disease.Therefore these results raise the fascinating possibility that chronic *H. pylori*-related inflam-mation is a significant cause of heart disease. However the authors

admit that much more work is needed before it is established that *H. pylori* actually causes such problems.

Who to focus our eradication strategy on

For the time being it is appropriate to precede stepwise, starting with patients who definitely need treatment and then treating their relatives who are likely to be at increased risk. As knowledge of the infection and diagnostic methods become available over the counter the public will test themselves using kits and request eradication therapy if they are infected. In the light of what we already know this is a reasonable request. If a mass eradication were to be undertaken it would seem advisable to test teenagers because these are past the age when most infection occurs and probably young enough to obtain maximum benefit, although we need more information on these points. It might be worthwhile treating the whole family in order to reduce the risk of re-infection.

Of course the whole scene will change again when immunization against *H. pylori* infection becomes available. It may then be possible to prevent an enormous amount of disease worldwide.

In the meantime the transmission of *H. pylori* can be diminished by improving sanitation and hygiene measures in developing countries. Unfortunately, unless we can overcome tribalism and famine this will not occur. At present the successful development of a vaccine seems more likely but it will then be a case of who pays for it, if anybody.

REFERENCES

1. Arvind AS, Cook RS, Tabaqchali S, Farthing MJ. One-minute endoscopy room test for *Campylobacter pylori* (letter). *Lancet* 1988; i: 704.
2. McNulty CA, Dent JC, Uff JS *et al*. Detection of *Campylobacter pylori* by the biopsy urease test: an assessment in 1445 patients. *Gut* 1989; **30**: 1058–1062.
3. Vaira D, Holton J. Urease tests for *Campylobacter pylori* detection (letter). *Am J Gastroenterol* 1989; **84**: 836–837.
4. Schrader JA, Peck HV, Notis WM *et al*. A role for culture in diagnosis of *Helicobacter pylori*-related gastric disease. *Am J Gastroenterol* 1993; **88**: 1729–1733.
5. Logan RPH, Walker MM, Misiewicz JJ *et al*. Changes in the intragastric distribution of *Helicobacter pylori* during treatment with omeprazole. *Gut* 1995; **36**: 12–16.

6. Kohli Y, Tanaka Y, Kato T, Ito S. Endoscopic diagnosis of *Helicobacter pylori* distribution in human gastric mucosa by phenol red dye spraying method. *Nippon Rinsho* 1993; **51**: 3182–3186.

7. Westblom TU, Phadnis S, Yang P, Czinn SJ. Diagnosis of *Helicobacter pylori* infection by means of a polymerase chain reaction assay for gastric juice aspirates. *Clin Infect Dis* 1993; **16**: 367–371.

8. Butcher GP, Ryder SD, Hughes SJ, *et al.* Use of an ammonia electrode for rapid quantification of *Helicobacter pylori* urease: its use in the endoscopy room and in the assessment of urease inhibition by bismuth subsalicylate. *Digestion* 1992; **53**: 142–148.

9. Edmonds PR, Carrozza MJ, Ruggiero FM *et al. Helicobacter (Campylobacter) pylori* in gastric brushing cytology. *Diag Cytopathol* 1992; **8**: 563–566.

10. Negrini R, Lisato L, Cavazzini L, *et al.* Monoclonal antibodies for specific immunoperoxidase detection of *Campylobacter pylori. Gastroenterology* 1989; **96**: 414–420.

11. Mathialagan R, Loizou S, Beales ILP *et al.* Who gets false-negative *H. pylori* (HP) ELISA results? (abstract). *Gut* 1994; **35**(suppl 5): S1.

12. Beales ILP, Crabtree JE, Covacci A, Calam J. Antibodies to CagA protein are associated with atrophic gastritis in *H. pylori* infection (abstract). *Gut* 1995; **35**(suppl 1): A45.

13. Kimura K, Ido I, Saifuku K *et al.* One-hour topical therapy for the eradication of *H. pylori* (abstract). *Am J Gastroenterol* 1994; **89**: 1403.

14. Bedwell J, Holton J, Vaira D *et al. In vitro* killing of *Helicobacter pylori* with photodynamic therapy (letter). *Lancet* 1990; **335**: 1287.

15. Chen M, Lee A, Hazell S. Immunisation against gastric *Helicobacter* infection in a mouse/*Helicobacter felis* model (letter). *Lancet* 1992; **339**: 1120–1121.

16. Doidge C, Crust I, Lee A *et al.* Therapeutic immunisation against *Helicobacter* infection (letter). *Lancet* 1994; **343**: 914–915.

17. Michetti P, Corthesy-Theulaz I, Vaney A-C *et al.* Prophylactic and therapeutic immunisation against *H. pylori felis* infection with *H. pylori* urease B subunit (abstract). *Am J Gastroenterol* 1994; **89**: 1343.

18. Mendall MA, Molineaux N, Levi J *et al.* Association of *H. pylori* with diminished adult height (abstract). *Gut* 1994; **35**(suppl 2): S4.

19. Raymond J, Bergeret M, Benhamou PH *et al.* A 2-year study of *Helicobacter pylori* in children. *J Clin Microbiol* 1994; **32**: 461–463.
20. Mendall MA, Goggin PM, Molineaux N *et al.* Relation of *Helicobacter pylori* infection and coronary heart disease. *Br Heart J* 1994; **71**: 437–439.
21. Patel P, Carrington D, Strachan DP *et al.* Fibrinogen: a link between chronic infection and coronary heart disease (letter). *Lancet* 1994; **343**: 1634–1635.

Index

References to figures are in **bold** type, references to tables are in *italics*